Sexplained....

The
uncensored
guide to sexual health

by
Helen Knox
RGN, Dip DN, FP & Adv FP Certs, FAETC
Clinical Nurse Specialist in Family Planning
and Sexual Health

KNOX PUBLISHING
Chiswick, London, UK

D0257537

First published in 1995

Enquiries to:-
Knox Publishing, PO Box 6969, Chiswick, London W4 3WX, England

This book is not intended to be a guide to the diagnosis, treatment or prognosis of any medical condition, whether physical or psychological. In case of illness, consult a Doctor.

© Helen Knox 1995

British Library Cataloguing in Publication Data.
A catalogue copy of this book is available from the British Library.

Knox, Helen
        Sexplained.... the uncensored guide to sexual health

        ISBN   0-9526224-0-8

Printed in Great Britain by Biddles Ltd.
Illustrations by Peter Gardiner
Cover, Page layout, Image setting and Graphics by Cy Pher, Islington, London.
Photography supplied by the National Medical Slidebank and Welcome Centre Medical Photo Library
Courtesy condom cartoon illustrations from :
1.   The 'getting it on' leaflet, designed in conjunction with FP Sales by Tim Davis MCSD
2.   The London Rubber Company

Acknowledgements

The idea for this book originated in the summer of 1992, after a teaching session, when Kathleen, an ex-prostitute said *"I never knew there was a bug out there which could make me unable to have a baby, with no signs or symptoms - more people should know what you have just told us. If I didn't know, in this job, how many others don't know? I would have made all my 'punters' wear condoms if I'd known"*. I thank her and wish her well.

In preparing this book, I have received much valuable advice from many people. I am very grateful to each of them for their continual support, encouragement, patience and time.

I do not know the names of many people who have read various portions 'along the way' - but they know who they are and I would like them to know that I am grateful for their assistance.

Others I do know and would like to express my appreciation to:
Mrs M Aird
Dr George Atallah M.B. Ch.B., D. Derm., D. Ven., Staff Physician in GU
    Medicine
Liz Clegg RGN, Dip.DN, Onc. N. Cert., Clinical Nurse Specialist - HIV
Mike Dibben
Sue Dibben SRN, NDN Cert., PWT
Mr C Emeribe
Annie Jansen-Pass
Vicky Padbury RGN, Adv. FP Cert., Clinical Nurse Specialist in Family
    Planning
Mrs Elizabeth Sebök RGN, SCM
Mr R Watt

The British Liver Trust - for permission to use their definition of 'cirrhosis'.
Dr K C Mohanty - for permission to use two of his photographs

Sharon, her friends and acquaintances in the 'sex industry'.

The Doctors, Nurses and Clerical Staff with whom I work in the Family Planning and Reproductive Health Service of West Lambeth, South London.

Finally, my Mother, for her endless support and encouragement.

H.K.

Introduction

Helen Knox trained as a Registered General Nurse at The Westminster Hospital, London. She worked as a Senior Staff Nurse at St Thomas' Hospital, London and as a District Nursing Sister in West London, before specialising in the field of Family Planning and Sexual Health. For the last 8 years she has been an Instructing Nurse and Clinical Nurse Specialist in this field, during which time she has worked throughout West, North West and South London. She has considerable experience teaching the subject to other professionals and the general public of all ages - male and female, young and 'not so young', in all sorts of unusual locations and situations. This book could not have been written without the teaching experience she gained at 'street level', the relaxed curiosity of the people she met along the way or the openness and honesty she encountered.

She was a finalist in the 1994 'Nursing Times /3M National Nursing Awards for Innovation in Nursing and Midwifery'. The comment made by the judges was that her work "in expanding the outreach work relating to Sexual Health and Family Planning advice was quite exceptional, and we hope very much that you will be able to continue to develop it".

This book provides comprehensive information about the many sexually transmitted infections and other sexual health matters in a simple, realistic, question and answer format. Some of the information may appear quite 'clinical' but it is necessary to explain the subject fully and provide a 'working guide' for all. It points to prevention and where applicable, cure. The layout of the book is designed to enable the reader to 'pick and choose' their way around 'short sharp answers' to questions, without becoming bored by the large areas of complex information and without trivialising the importance of each topic.

In no way does this book intend to encourage anyone to do anything except 'keep safe'! It appreciates that many activities occur at all sorts of ages, by all sorts of people, in all sorts of ways and that you cannot tell by looking at someone if they have any infections. It is written from a UK perspective and acknowledges that some of the information on services available, is more appropriate to urban than rural areas, where services are further afield and less 'anonymous' or where different services are available in different countries.

Although some people may not like some of the contents of this book (or feel that this may not be suitable for young people), it is better to give full and accurate information on subjects they ask about, than to refuse to answer openly or fully from ignorance or embarrassment - perhaps then leaving people 'at risk'!

A lot of time and research about the frequency of the less openly discussed activities has gone into the decision about inclusion of information. It is felt that leaving anything out on the grounds of any 'taboo' would be wrong and not educate properly about the serious risks to sexual health or guide to the prevention of infection.

No-one wants HIV. HIV has brought the subject of sexual health more into the open, although it cannot be seen. No-one wants any of the infections mentioned in this book, all of which are very common, many of which can be seen. They are nearly all caught the same way - through sex!

The general public do not, on the whole, get to see the reality of what is seen in clinics. Colour pictures are included because during her hundreds of teaching sessions, Helen has found that it is those which leave the lasting impression about the seriousness of the conditions. Although some people may have found them horrible to look at, they have appreciated the honesty and chance to see what they could only previously imagine. The large majority wanted their friends and relatives to see the reality of what can happen. They are not used to shock but to inform, educate, generate discussion, thought and self respect. Many people wished they had been shown similar material when they were much younger.

The book points out that hepatitis is much easier to catch than HIV and explains this subject in depth. The section on **'What *is* safer sex?'** re-assesses risk behaviour and aims to protect people from *all* sexually transmitted infections, **not just HIV** - and explains that many practices considered 'safe' against HIV are, in fact, unsafe against many others, if they are present.

It may not be a **'coffee table book'**, but perhaps it should be! - to generate discussion and greater awareness of these 'facts of life'.

It is hoped that this guide will prove interesting, educational and helpful to all who read it.

Contents

Meaning of Some Words Used in this Book

adhesions	-	where two normally separate surfaces stick together - usually happens as the result of scarring after inflammation
AIDS	-	acquired immune deficiency syndrome
anal	-	of the back passage
ampoule	-	sealed glass capsule, containing sterile dose of drug in solution or sterile water for injection
back passage	-	anus and rectum
burrows	-	little tracks or 'tunnels'
cervix	-	neck of the womb or 'uterus'
colposcopy	-	is when the neck of the womb is viewed by a Doctor or Nurse with a special magnifying instrument which looks like a pair of binoculars (which stays outside the woman). They look to see the extent of the unusual cell pattern and if necessary, give treatment
down below	-	genital area, 'private area'
ejaculation	-	the act of discharging semen ('cumming') at orgasm or sexual climax
erection	-	'hard on' or sexually active state of the penis when enlarged and rigid
faeces	-	the body waste which is passed through the back passage (anus)
fallopian tubes	-	the pair of tubes which lead from the uterus (womb) to the ovaries - where the egg and sperm meet, start to divide and multiply, before travelling back towards the womb to implant and grow into a baby
fertility	-	being able to make a baby
FP	-	family planning
genital	-	relates to the reproductive organs
genitalia	-	external reproductive organs - in this context (e.g.penis, labia-'lips down below', vaginal entrance etc.)
glands	-	parts of the body which produce special fluids
glans	-	glans penis - the acorn shaped end of the man's penis or woman's clitoris
GUM	-	genito - urinary medicine
HIV	-	human immunodeficiency virus
hormone	-	a substance made in one part of the body which travels via the bloodstream to affect another part of the body
HPV	-	human papilloma virus
HSV	-	herpes simplex virus
impotence	-	the inability to get and keep an erection of the penis
infertility	-	being unable to make a baby
irritable bowel syndrome	-	'spastic colon' or alternating and recurrent syndrome abdominal pain causing constipation and diarrhoea in the absence of ill health

IUD	-	it is usually a small plastic device with copper and/or silver wrapped around it to prevent pregnancy when inserted into the womb - also known as an intra-uterine device or 'coil'
IUS	-	or 'intra-uterine system' is a new (1995 UK launch) hormone releasing 'coil' - similar to 'coil'/IUD above, but instead of copper and/or silver, it has the hormone 'progestogen' wrapped around it which is slowly released into the woman's body - prevents pregnancy and reduces excess menstrual bleeding when fitted
menstruation	-	woman's 'menses', 'period', 'monthly', 'the curse' etc. - when the lining of the womb sheds away if no pregnancy has occurred that month or 'cycle'
oral	-	of the mouth
ovulation	-	when a woman's ovary releases an egg
pre-conceptual	-	before conception - when planning a baby
premature ejaculation	-	not being able to control ejaculation ('cumming') for long after sex starts
sex worker	-	'prostitute'
STD	-	sexually transmitted disease (V.D.)
suppresses	-	temporarily stops
swab	-	a pad of cotton wool wrapped tightly around a wooden or plastic stick. It is wiped through a discharge, so that a sample can be collected for the laboratory to check which germs are present
taboo	-	generally disapproved of
TSS	-	toxic shock syndrome
tubes	-	fallopian tubes
ultrasound	-	ultrasonic waves - sound waves which can't be heard but with the help of a special machine, produce pictures of inside the body
universal precautions	-	standard or routine precautions which are understood and used by all 'healthcare professionals', to prevent infection and/or cross infection
unprotected sex	-	sex without protection against pregnancy or germs
VD	-	venereal disease - disease which is transmitted by sex
withdrawal	-	here, it means the removal of the penis during sex - before ejaculation occurs

Section 1

Services available to men and women

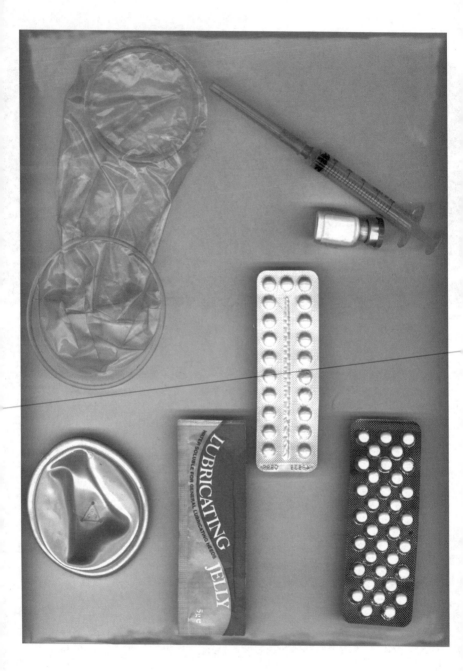

What is contraception?
* it is a method used by men or women to stop a pregnancy occurring

Where can I get contraception?
it is available from:
* any Family Planning or Reproductive Health Clinic
* most family Doctors (GP's)
* within some GUM clinics (genito-urinary medicine, also known as STD or 'sexually transmitted disease' clinics) at special times
* from some privately run clinics e.g. Marie Stopes International, Pregnancy Advisory Service and British Pregnancy Advisory Service
* in many areas there are special clinics for 'young people' (e.g. 'Brook' in the UK, which see people under the age of 25 years)

Do I have to be married or planning a family to go to a Family Planning Clinic?
* no, they care for young and old, male and female, married or single
* there are no age limits and there is no judgement of what you tell them, so don't feel shy

Do they need to see any identification of who I am?
* no, they accept what you tell them

How old do I have to be to be seen?
* any age - even if you are under 16

* generally, you do not have to take your Mum or other adult with you

If I am under the legal age of consent, won't they think I'm a 'bad' person for going to see them for help?
* no, they will not
* they are not there to judge you
* they respect your choice and the maturity which prompted you to seek advice

Do they contact any 'authority' like the police, social workers, parents, guardians, hostel workers etc.?
* no-one is contacted without your permission
* their concern is only for YOU

Will they 'lecture' me?
* no, what you do and how you do it is your business
* any questions you may have about 'safer sex' or safer injecting of drugs can be asked freely of the Nurse or Doctor

So, if I inject drugs, can I still come to the clinic?
* yes

Will they tell my Doctor if I go to a clinic?
* no, the service is strictly confidential and your Doctor is only contacted with your permission, even though some clinics like to encourage you to let them write to your GP
* always remember, the choice is yours

Sexplained © 1995 Helen Knox

How can I be sure?
- if you are THAT worried, you can give only a contact address, but make sure it is a reliable means by which to contact you, in case you need treatment and do not realise it

Am I bound to return to the same clinic if I start to go?
- no, you are not
- if you ask, they can write a transfer note for you to take to another clinic, or Doctor, about any treatments or methods you are using
- it is sensible to stay with one provider of care, so that there is continuity of medical care
- but the choice is yours

Won't they laugh at me for my problems?
- no
- they are only interested in helping you as much as you wish

What does a Family Planning Clinic offer?
   Family Planning Clinics offer all methods of contraception, free - i.e: -
- the combined oral contraceptive pill (the pill)
- the progesterone only pill (mini pill)
- the coil/IUD (intra-uterine contraceptive device)
- the combination IUS - intra-uterine system - a coil with the hormone progesterone attached. (a new method which was launched in 1995)
- the Dutch cap/diaphragm (which fits the length of the vagina and covers the cervix or 'neck of the womb')
- the cervical cap (a cap which just fits over the cervix or 'neck of the womb')
- emergency contraception
- injectable contraception
- male and female condoms (either for contraception or in addition to another contraceptive method - for 'safer sex')
- advice on 'natural' family planning (safe period) or referral to a specialist 'teacher' of this method
- Norplant, a 5 year contraceptive implant (or referral to a specialist centre to have it fitted)
- referral for male sterilization (vasectomy)
- referral for female sterilization

Do they offer anything else?
   they also offer:
- free pregnancy testing
- pre-conceptual advice
- advice and counselling about rape, impotence, premature ejaculation, and many other sexual worries
- referral for unwanted pregnancy counselling
- post-abortion support and counselling
- for women of all ages, they will check your breasts (if you want) and teach you how to be 'breast aware'
- they do cervical ('pap') smear tests for women of all ages

- ❖ hysterectomy advice and support
- ❖ menopause advice/support and referral for HRT (hormone replacement therapy)
- ❖ relationship counselling
- ❖ they may check blood for rubella (German measles), sickle cell and thalassaemia
- ❖ there are blood pressure and weight checks for both men and women
- ❖ advice on testicular health and 'testicular self-examination' techniques
- ❖ male attendees are increasing and often want to talk their problems through with people who will give them time and listen - so don't feel that you or your friends will be the first
- ❖ many young men find the idea of going to a clinic and talking to people off-putting, but once they have been they wish they had taken the opportunity before
- ❖ there are male Doctors at some clinics if you would prefer to talk to a male
- ❖ Family Planning clinics are NOT 'women only' clinics
- ❖ but some areas have started specific clinics only for men

Are the Doctors male or female?
- ❖ the Doctors are usually female in the clinics
- ❖ if you require a male Doctor, enquire at reception

Do they have any male Doctors?
- ❖ yes, they do occasionally, but they are aware that many men

and women prefer female Doctors
- ❖ if this is your preference, just say
- ❖ however, they are all specialists in Family Planning with considerable medical experience in this field

How much does it cost?
- ❖ nothing - all the NHS services and supplies are FREE in the UK

women
What does having an 'internal' involve?
- ❖ first, this is not a 'must' at your first visit or before you get contraception
- ❖ it may only be necessary if you, yourself have any health concerns
- ❖ it is a gentle examination by a Doctor of your 'private' area (vaginal examination)
- ❖ you may find the thought of this embarrassing at your first visit, but the doctor only wants to make sure that everything is alright with you
- ❖ they may, or may not, suggest using a special instrument, called a speculum
- ❖ this enables the Doctor to look inside your vagina and check that the cervix (neck of the womb) is healthy
- ❖ Doctors appreciate that some women find this embarrassing but it is the only way to check if you really are alright
- ❖ there is often a Nurse with you to reassure you and hold your hand - if there is not and you would like one to be there, just ask
- ❖ it really is far better to 'pluck up

Sexplained © 1995 Helen Knox

the courage' and be sure you are alright, than to neglect your health from embarrassment

Does it hurt?
* no, it does not
* it may be uncomfortable
* but the more relaxed you are the more comfortable it is
* afterwards many people say "is that it? I didn't feel a thing - I don't know why I was so frightened."

Do I HAVE to have one?
* no, but it is sometimes advised in your best health interests. However, the ultimate decision is yours

What is a smear test?
* this is when the neck of the womb is wiped with a special instrument called a 'spatula'
* the spatula is then wiped across a piece of glass, which is then 'fixed' with a special solution and sent to the laboratory
* the laboratory checks the sample to see if any of the cells or covering of the cervix (neck of the womb) have changed from the normal pattern
* sometimes 'abnormal' cells are noticed, which can gradually lead to 'pre-cancer' of the cervix, if they are not treated
* and if 'pre-cancer' is left untreated it can lead to 'cancer of the cervix', womb and travel into the rest of the body
* treatment is now easy, quick and

highly successful

Why should I have a smear test?
* the aim is to save you any further trouble in the years to come and to look after your future health

Do I have to have a smear test?
* no
* the ultimate decision is yours

men and women
Can I just go to the clinic for condoms?
* yes, and they are free
* they will usually ask for minimal information in the clinics, but some areas offer free condoms at "condom supply points" where no questions are asked

Where can I find these "condom supply points"?
* each area is different but if you ring your local hospital and ask for the Family Planning Office, they should be able to tell you what your area offers
* BUT condoms are also available at all Family Planning Clinics in the country - FREE

Why is it called a clinic when I'm not ill?
* good question!
* the word clinic means 'a centre at which advice and assistance in matters of health, hygiene, maternity etc. are given'

men or women

If I have or have had many partners am I still welcome?

❖ yes, you are

❖ they will not judge your lifestyle or lecture you in any way

What may a clinic need from me?
women

❖ you will always be asked to give the date of the FIRST day of your last 'period'

❖ if that is 'today' then say that, otherwise try and work out the date beforehand

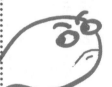

❖ likewise, if you want a pregnancy test, they need something to test! - so take a sample of urine ('wee') you pass that day, for testing

❖ the first 'wee' is the most concentrated - but other samples can still give an accurate result

❖ sometimes you may be asked to repeat the test later with an early morning/first specimen

❖ you don't need a special container - a clean jar or bottle will do and only a few drops are needed.

What is the 'morning after pill'?
* it is what is now called 'emergency contraception'

OK! So what is 'emergency contraception'?
* it is four special hormone pills, the first two should be taken WITHIN 72 hours (3 days) of unprotected sex. The second two, exactly 12 hours later
* both doses should be taken after food has been eaten
* the treatment is available for those who have either had unprotected sex or those who have had an 'accident' with their chosen method of contraception
* if you miss the 72 hours don't panic, because an 'emergency coil/IUD' can be fitted into the womb up to 5 days after unprotected sex, by a specially trained Family Planning Doctor
* both of these methods alter the conditions inside the womb to prevent an unplanned pregnancy

Can I take a friend or an interpreter with me?
* yes and having company can make you less nervous!
* some clinics have interpreters but it helps the clinic staff, too, if English is not your first language

Will they show me how to use whatever they give me?
* yes
* they teach you how to use your contraceptive method(s) properly and make sure you understand what to do if things go wrong
* if you are ever in any doubt, PLEASE ASK FOR HELP
* you do not need an appointment to ask for help
* alternatively you could phone for advice, when the clinic is open

Are there any 'help-lines' I can ring for advice?
* you can ring any Family Planning Clinic and ask to speak to a Doctor or Nurse
* details of clinics can be found in the 'phone book' or at the library
* you can ring and ask to speak to your GP or Practice Nurse
* your Pharmacist (chemist) can help you
* general information is available from the Family Planning Association in London and they can also tell you about clinics available throughout the country. Their number is:-
  0171-636-7866
* you can also see *any* GP in the country who offers contraceptive services - even if they are not your own GP

Is there anything I should be aware of?

- GUM is the new name for STD clinic
- they were previously known as 'special' or 'VD' clinics
- they are usually open Monday to Friday, 9 am to 5 pm - but ring your local hospital, to check their opening times and whether they run an appointment, a 'walk-in' clinic or both services
- you are seen on the day you decide to attend
- sometimes you may have to wait if they are very busy and also because they diagnose some tests results 'on the spot' which takes time
- they then give you the correct treatment for your specific infection
- you do not need to be referred to this clinic by your GP - you can walk in and ask to be seen
- some have a special 'fast lane'- a prioritised and speedy walk-in service for male and female 'sex workers'

What else is available?

- all counselling and medication is FREE
- if you are on 'income support' fares are reimbursed
- Hepatitis B vaccination is available - it is usually 3 injections over 7 months
- 'emergency contraceptive pills' are available up to 72 hours after unprotected sex, at some GUM/STD Clinics
- emergency IUD's are not usually inserted in GUM/STD clinics, although they may be willing to refer you to a Family Planning Clinic for one - but if you have a pelvic infection at the time, a coil/IUD is not advised
- they do cervical smear tests and if there are abnormalities further tests and treatment can also be done quickly and accurately in this department
- if they are not the right department for your problem, they can immediately refer you to the correct department in the hospital

Is everything confidential?

- their service is totally confidential - by law
- they won't tell you what your partner has, nor will they tell your partner what you have unless you request their help and intervention
- likewise, they won't inform your GP of anything unless you give your permission

If they keep notes on me, what information do they need?

- they ask for a name and date of birth (preferably your own, but this is not essential)

Sexplained © 1995 Helen Knox

- it is just to 'cross reference' the clinic number used for filing
- a 'contact address' may be requested, but if you prefer not to give an address, they will not turn you away and you will still be treated
- whatever you tell them, though, make sure it is something you will easily remember for your return visit(s)
- they can then find your correct notes and treatment record quickly and easily

Who works there?

- Doctors, Nurses and Clerical staff 'Health Advisors', who explain about each infection and help you understand what has to be done to make you better
- a psycho-sexual counsellor (someone to talk sexual problems through with) often works in the GUM/STD department

How can I help the staff?

- **MEN** can help by not passing urine for 3 - 4 hours before any swabs or specimens are taken, to ensure better results
- **WOMEN** can help by working out the date of the <u>first day</u> of your last period in advance, as this will always be asked for
- it is OK to have a period when you attend but they are unlikely to do a 'smear test' or 'colposcopy' on those days and may ask you to return, but other tests can be carried out

What is a 'contact slip' and why do some people get one?

- a 'contact slip' is a specially coded piece of paper which tells another Doctor which infection(s), in particular, they should check for
- if you are given one they will ask you to give it to your sexual partner or partners
- they can then take it into any GUM/STD clinic in the country and be correctly examined and treated
- using it is an important way you can help the Doctors and avoid re-infection

Can I have an HIV test at a GUM/STD clinic?

- totally confidential HIV counselling and testing are available
- it is available by appointment for 'same day results' in a lot of clinics
- treatment is available for those who are 'HIV antibody positive' with referral to other hospital departments, including dental, community and social care, if desired
- some clinics give general test results over the phone, but NOT HIV test results

Can I take my children with me?

- they are not places designed for children, but they can go with you

General information

* you will not shock anyone working in these clinics so do not feel shy to answer all questions openly and honestly
* most things are treatable - so go early and get any problems sorted out - don't let anything go on or get worse, due to your embarrassment
* if you think you have an infection, don't take your friend's medication or some you have 'hanging around'
* visit the clinic to get the correct 'in date' medication and proper diagnosis of what YOU have got
* if you notice any abnormal lumps, bumps, blisters or discharges, particularly in your 'private' area -
* it is far better to go along and get checked
* being told there is nothing wrong is better than ignoring something because you are embarrassed, which might cause problems later on and may have been cured quite simply
* it is sensible for everyone to have a check up, from time to time
* germs can spread genitally ('down below') or orally (by mouth), so the same protection is necessary when practicing oral sex as penetrative sex (vaginal or anal).
* See p.59 'What *is* safer sex?'

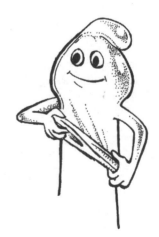

Section 2

Things you should know but may not have been told

Other name:
❖ B.V.

Where does it come from?
❖ the main causes are 'gardnerella' and 'anaerobic vaginosis'
❖ at present it is uncertain whether they are sexually transmitted

How do I get it?
❖ it is the result of an imbalance of the conditions in the vagina
❖ it is considered, by some, to be a sexually transmitted infection
❖ some women notice a regular pattern to the increase and decrease of their symptoms - due to changing hormone levels throughout their menstrual cycle
❖ the vaginal conditions after termination of pregnancy (abortion), hysterectomy (removal of the womb) or other gynaecological treatment can become imbalanced and BV can then develop

What might I notice?
women
❖ you will probably notice an increase in vaginal secretion
❖ the discharge often looks like a runny, grey coloured, 'flour paste' which will probably smell 'fishy'
❖ you will probably feel embarrassed by the odour - which will often 'show up', or smell worse, when you have sex
❖ your partner may notice it before you do
❖ you may not notice anything or be bothered by the discharge
❖ there may be slight itching and inflammation 'down below'
men
❖ you may notice nothing at all
❖ sometimes the head of your penis may be inflamed and sore

What tests would I have?
❖ a swab (sample taken by wiping a special cotton wool bud through the discharge) would be taken and viewed under a microscope

What treatment is there, if I have B.V.?
❖ antibiotics - the course must be taken properly and no alcohol taken whilst on these tablets - they don't mix and would probably make you sick

What should I do after I finish the treatment?
❖ return to normal
❖ if you are someone who keeps getting these attacks, you may try using condoms, to prevent the possibility of re-infection
❖ your partner should be tested and treated
❖ the symptoms can come in women who are not sexually active
❖ it seems to recur of its own accord in many people, so different treatments may be suggested

What about my partner?
❖ in persistent cases, they should be checked at an STD clinic even if they do not have any symptoms

What about sex?
* be advised by the Doctor treating you
* see p.59 'What *is* safer sex?'

because of the associated odour
* pregnant women with BV are more at risk of miscarriage or giving birth prematurely

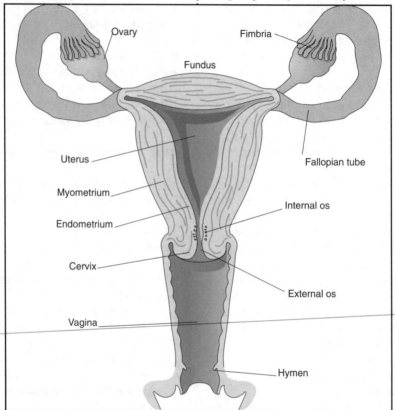

Ovary
Fimbria
Fundus
Uterus
Fallopian tube
Myometrium
Endometrium
Internal os
Cervix
External os
Vagina
Hymen

What about oral sex, anal sex and condoms?
* see p.59 'What *is* safer sex?'

What complications can come from having B.V?
* it can be a contributing factor in pelvic inflammatory disease (see PID)
* for many women with recurrent infection - there can be relationship and sexual problems

How can I avoid getting it?
* the reason for its occurrence is not fully understood but the use of condoms may help to prevent recurrence
* it is a common cause of vaginal discharge in developed countries
* it can develop in women who are not sexually active
* in some women, it goes away on its own

(for men only)
Other names:
- balanoposthitis
- inflammation of the head of the penis (balanitis)
- inflammation of the foreskin (posthitis)

Where does it come from?
- 'thrush' (see 'thrush' section)
- poor personal hygiene - the foreskin must be pulled back and the area underneath washed every day
- trauma or accidental damage to the penis
- diabetes
- allergy to drugs or contraceptive spermicide
- long foreskin
- tight foreskin
- reaction to antiseptics or disinfectants
- an illness which can be caused by chlamydia called Reiter's disease
- rarely, moist shiny red patches on the tip of the penis or under the foreskin are pre-malignant (pre-cancerous) so it is important to be checked properly

How do I get balanitis?
- some causes are sexually transmitted but many are not (see above)

How long does balanitis take to show?
- variable lengths of time - it depends upon the cause

What might I notice?
you may notice one or more of the following on your penis:
- spots or a rash
- redness
- itching
- discomfort and/or pain
- discharge
- pain during sex
- swelling, which may be fluid filled and make it difficult to pull back the foreskin, which may become tight
- cracks may appear on the skin of the penis
- you may have pain or experience difficulty in passing urine

What tests would I have?
- swabs (sample taken by wiping a special cotton wool bud through the discharge) would be taken and sent to the laboratory
- some specimens are viewed in the GUM/STD clinic, at the time of your visit

What treatment is there, if I have balanitis?
- if your cause is from an infection you will be given the appropriate antibiotic or cream
- if the foreskin will pull back (retract), bathing the area four times a day, for 5 - 10 minutes in a salt-water solution (one heaped tablespoonful of salt to one pint of warm water) will be of great comfort
- if the foreskin does not pull back (retract) special cleaning techniques are usually taught -

Sexplained © 1995 Helen Knox

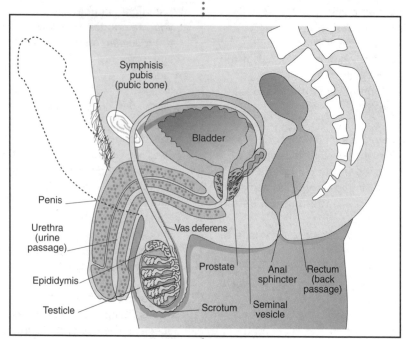

using a syringe (without a needle attached!) to irrigate the sore areas with the salt water solution
* some men are advised to have a circumcision (surgical removal of the foreskin), if the trouble persists

What should I do after I finish the treatment?
* be advised by the Doctor treating you as it will depend upon the cause

What about my partner?
* it is wise for them to be tested and treated if necessary

What about sex, oral sex, anal sex and condoms?
* it is wise to avoid sex whilst you are being treated
* see p.59 **'What *is* safer sex?'**

What complications can come from having balanitis?
* if your cause is sexually transmitted - see the section on the particular infection
* 'phimosis' or narrowing of the foreskin may occur after repeated injury
* the foreskin may require surgical removal (circumcision), if the condition is severe

How can I avoid getting balanitis?
* good personal hygiene
* avoid sexually transmitted infections by wearing a condom each time you have sex
* the area in question is a sensitive

one, so treat it gently

❖ if you notice discomfort which is not from a sexually transmitted infection, try to work out what has caused it, to avoid repeat attacks

❖ be aware of your health and seek medical attention before minor conditions get worse

❖ this condition is very common so don't be shy when talking to a Doctor about it further

❖ see p.59 **'What *is* safer sex?'**

Sexplained © 1995 Helen Knox

(pronounced 'cla - mi -dea')

Where does it come from?

❖ it comes from a germ or bacterium called 'chlamydia trachomatis'

How do I get chlamydia?

❖ it is sexually transmitted

How long does chlamydia take to show?

❖ usually from about 1 - 2 weeks
❖ BUT it can 'lie dormant' (sleeping) causing no problems and showing no signs for many years - in both men and women

What might I notice?

you may notice one or more of the following:

women -

❖ vaginal discharge
❖ pain on passing urine
❖ abdominal pain
❖ pain with sex
❖ bleeding between periods
❖ bleeding after sex
❖ heavier than usual periods
❖ pain or cramps in the stomach or lower back - particularly after sex
 but
❖ **70%** of **women** have **no symptoms**

men -

❖ discharge from the tip of the penis
❖ pain on passing urine
❖ itching around the opening of the penis
❖ pain or swelling of the testicles

 but
❖ 25% of **men** have **no symptoms**

babies -

❖ can contract it via vaginal (normal) delivery if the Mother has it
❖ it shows as 'sticky eye' and conjunctivitis (inflammation) of the eye
❖ this is becoming more common and the detection of chlamydia is improving

What tests would I have?

❖ special 'swab' test, but it takes 1 - 2 weeks for the results to grow and show in the laboratory, hence the delay

What treatment is there, if I have chlamydia?

❖ antibiotic tablets
❖ the course of tablets must be completed, even if you feel better, or the infection will return
❖ no alcohol should be taken whilst taking them

What should I do after I finish the treatment?

❖ your Doctor or GUM/STD clinic may suggest that you return to see them
❖ be advised by whoever treats you

What about my partner?

❖ your partner(s) should be checked for any infections at a GUM/STD clinic as soon as possible and treated

What about sex?

❖ this is a **very important** question - you should have **no oral or penetrative sex for two weeks until all the chlamydia has been cleared and until you have been re-checked or given the o.k. by the Doctor treating you**

❖ even sex with a condom is **unacceptable** in case of failure or from the germ also being present in the bladder, throat etc.

What about oral sex, anal sex and condoms?

❖ avoid this whilst having treatment see p.59 **'What *is* safer sex?'**

What complications can come from having chlamydia?

women

❖ if chlamydia is not treated, the fallopian tubes may become inflamed and may block, the ovaries and womb may become involved, causing abdominal pain, leaving P.I.D. - pelvic inflammatory disease

❖ there may be an increased risk of ectopic (tubal) pregnancy

❖ there may be an increased danger of infertility (being unable to have a baby)

men

❖ the 'tubes' in the man can become inflamed, scarred or blocked which may increase the risk of infertility

How can I avoid getting chlamydia?

❖ never assume that a 'clean looking' person is clear of infection

❖ see p.59 **"What *is* safer sex?"**

Sexplained © 1995 Helen Knox

(more common in women)

Other names:
- inflammation of the bladder and urine passage
- 'honeymoon cystitis'

Where does it come from?
there are several causes:
- it is very common in sexually active women
- germs from the bowel may spread towards the vagina and urethra (urine passage) during sex, then climb up the short urine passage and multiply rapidly in the bladder, causing irritation and inflammation
- the germs of some sexually transmitted infections can get into the bladder this way and cause other problems (e.g. 'chlamydia')
- some women are allergic to scented soaps and vaginal deodorants which may cause problems
- tight trousers, tights and nylon underwear all make the 'private area' more moist and 'sweaty', giving germs the opportunity to multiply and cause problems
- 'holding on' for a 'wee' gives time for germs to multiply in the bladder before being 'flushed out' men have a much longer urine passage and germs have further to climb to the bladder, which takes them longer
- children and men rarely get it cystitis

How do I get cystitis?
- apart from the cystitis related directly to sexually transmitted infections, it can come from any of the above causes
- it is not a sexually transmitted infection although the delicate urine passage may be 'bruised' during sex which then makes it uncomfortable to pass urine ('wee')
- passing urine then gets 'put off', which gives germs time to multiply
- when using the cap or diaphragm for contraception, there may be added pressure against the vaginal and bladder walls, which can 'trap' urine in the bladder
- if you do not remember to empty your bladder before and after sex, the urine has the opportunity to 'stagnate' and germs may then multiply. This may lead to cystitis

How long does it take to show?
- it often starts within a few hours, or days, of whatever has triggered it off

What might I notice?
- there is often a burning or stinging pain on passing urine ('weeing')
- you may need to pass urine more often or feel as if you are 'bursting to go', but when you do, there may be very little urine to pass!
- **but** if you notice temperature, low back pain, with pain and/or bleeding on passing urine - you need to see a Doctor as soon as

possible, as the infection may have moved further up towards your kidneys and may be causing 'pyelonephritis' (inflammation of part of the kidney)

❖ this could lead to scarring of the kidneys

What tests would I have?

❖ a urine specimen would be sent to the laboratory if you go to see your Doctor, Family Planning Clinic or GUM/STD Clinic

What treatment is there if I have cystitis?

❖ normally the urine is slightly 'acid', but with cystitis it may be made very 'acid' by the germs, so treatment aims to reduce these high acid levels

❖ if you are pregnant, consult your Doctor and do not try 'home treatments' without their approval

❖ for non-pregnant women - your Doctor or GUM/STD clinic would give you antibiotics if you need them

❖ but many women prefer to try other methods first, as antibiotics can lead to 'thrush' - which can be extremely uncomfortable, too!

home treatments include:-

❖ drinking lots of water, lemon barley water, cranberry juice, orange squash, or mineral water will help to keep the bladder and kidneys 'well flushed' and gradually ease the pain - 1 pint straight away then half-a-pint, every 20 to 30 minutes for three to four hours

❖ a teaspoonful of bicarbonate of soda (to neutralize the acid) in your drink, every two hours will reduce the symptoms and pain quite quickly

❖ if you have heart or blood pressure problems you should discuss it with your Doctor first

❖ you may like to take mild pain killers (ask your Pharmacist's advice, if you are unsure)

❖ you may get so much pain that you simply can't pass urine without crying - if so, you may find it comfortable to pass urine in a warm bath (but clean the bath thoroughly, before and after use, especially if it is shared with others)

❖ lying down and cuddling a hot water bottle may help

What should I do after I finish the treatment?

❖ you should continue to drink plenty of fluid, regularly - approximately 4 pints a day (unless you are on 'restricted fluid intake' for a medical reason) to keep your kidneys and bladder 'well flushed'

What about my partner?

❖ they should be checked in case your infection has been sexually transmitted

What about sex?

❖ you can have sex when you feel comfortable enough

Sexplained © 1995 Helen Knox

What about oral sex, anal sex and condoms?

❖ see p.59 **'What *is* safer sex?'**

What complications can come from having cystitis?

❖ there are not usually long term complications from cystitis

❖ inflammation of the kidneys (pyelonephritis) can lead to scarring (damage from the inflamed surfaces sticking together)

❖ in pregnant women however, it should be treated by a Doctor each time as cystitis can lead to an increased risk of miscarriage, premature (early) delivery and to having a baby which is 'small for dates'

How can I avoid getting it?

❖ see 'Where does it come from?' and avoid as many of those as possible

❖ keep drinking plenty of fluid - 4 pints a day

❖ pass urine before and after sex

❖ you and your partner should wash 'down below' before and after sex always wipe 'from front to back' - especially after opening your bowels, to avoid moving bowel germs forward (towards the urine passage), where they could easily climb into the bladder and cause cystitis

❖ wash your 'private area' with soap and water, (using a special flannel used only for this purpose) and rinse with luke-warm water, after opening your bowels

❖ wear stockings rather than tights

❖ avoid using bubble bath or shampoo in the bath if you notice a link with attacks of cystitis

❖ notice whether perfumed or even perfume free soaps bring on an attack and if so, avoid them

❖ avoid food or drink which 'trigger' an attack i.e. tea, coffee, alcohol or foods like asparagus, which make the urine 'more acid'

Other name:
- condylomata acuminata

Where do they come from?
- they come from a virus called 'Human Papilloma Virus' (HPV)
- there are approximately 73 different varieties - some cause warts on other parts of the body and some just in the genital area

How do I get them?
- close physical or sexual contact

How long do they it take to show?
- any time from 3 to 18 months

What might I notice?
- they can 'lie dormant' (sleeping) and you may not notice anything yourself
- they may only be found when a partner notices that they have them or they are told at another routine check-up (e.g. smear test)
- there may be general itching and inflammation 'down below' or around the 'back passage'
- there may be tenderness
- there may be obviously visible warts or 'cauliflower like' clusters of warts
- there may be a feeling of 'lumps' growing on the skin
- there may be alteration in the strength and direction of your urine stream ('wee')

What tests would I have?
- a Doctor would look at the warts, perhaps with a magnifying glass under a good light
- for women, smear tests may show the presence of wart virus at the neck of the womb
- sometimes women may be asked to have a 'colposcopy' at the hospital, when the neck of the womb is viewed with a special magnifying glass

What treatment is there, if I have them?
men and women
- some warts are painted with special medicine
- others have to be frozen off
- or burnt off under local anaesthetic
- some of the treatments can take several weeks and involve many visits to the clinic
women
- some warts, on the neck of the womb, have to be treated by various minor surgical measures

What should I do after I finish the treatment?
- be guided by the Doctor treating you

What about my partner?
- however much you may be embarrassed, it is important to tell your partner
- they should be checked at a GUM/STD clinic, even if no warts can be seen
- **for women,** regular cervical smear tests are also strongly advised
- these should be yearly for 3 years, then if clear, every 3 years

What about sex?

❖ there is a risk of passing on the virus at any time but the most likely time is whilst warts are present, until the 'all clear' is given by the Doctor treating you, usually about 3 - 6 months after completion of the treatment

❖ take the advice of the Doctor treating you

❖ some Doctors advise abstaining (no sex or even masturbation) until the treatment is finished, as friction spreads warts

What about oral sex, anal sex and condoms?

❖ warts can be passed by oral or anal sex, so it is essential to use condoms

❖ see p.59 **'What *is* safer sex?'**

What complications can come from having them?

❖ four varieties of wart virus (HPV 16, 18, 31 and 34) are often found in cervical abnormalities, including pre-cancerous changes, when combined with other risk factors

❖ babies of women with genital wart virus are at risk of contracting the virus during birth

❖ genital warts can return

❖ if they are in the urine passage, the urine flow may be altered

❖ they may become infected and bleed, making them painful and cause discomfort

❖ they may spread around the warm moist 'private area' and cause great distress

How can I avoid getting them?

❖ the virus can lie dormant (sleeping) for many months, so the risk is there for most people

❖ don't share towels or underwear

❖ see p.59 **'What *is* safer sex?'**

Gonorrhoea

Other name:
 ❖ 'the clap' or 'the drip'

Where does it come from?
 ❖ it comes from a bacterium or germ (neisseria gonorrhoeae) which likes to live in warm moist areas of the body

How do I get gonorrhoea?
 ❖ it is sexually transmitted

How long does gonorrhoea take to show?
 ❖ usually 2 - 10 days after contact with the infection

What might I notice?
 there may be one or more of the following:-
 <u>*women may notice*</u>
 ❖ an unusual vaginal discharge which may increase, may become thin and watery, yellow or greenish
 ❖ there may be a burning sensation when you are passing urine
 ❖ there may be pain in the abdomen (just below your stomach)
 <u>**BUT**</u>
 ❖ **2 out of 3 women with gonorrhoea show no signs or symptoms!**
 <u>*men may notice*</u>
 ❖ a burning pain on passing urine
 ❖ yellow discharge from the penis
 ❖ tenderness in the testicles
 ❖ sometimes there may be irritation or discharge from the anus (opening to back passage)
 <u>**BUT**</u>

❖ **1 out of 10 men with gonorrhoea show no signs or symptoms!**

What tests would I have?
 ❖ laboratory test in a GUM/STD clinic, where the sample is viewed 'on the spot'

What treatment is there, if I have gonorrhoea?
 ❖ antibiotics
 ❖ the full course of treatment has to be taken to ensure a cure

What should I do after I finish the treatment?
 ❖ it is essential that you return to the clinic for a check-up after the treatment has finished, to make sure that all the gonorrhoea has gone
 ❖ women should also attend for smears tests as instructed

What about my partner?
 ❖ it is important that you contact them, as many people have gonorrhoea without realising and it needs treatment
 ❖ they should be seen at a GUM/STD clinic, tested and treated as necessary

What about sex?
 ❖ it is essential not to have sex with anyone until you have been advised that it is safe to resume - and until your partner has been cleared of the infection, too
 ❖ otherwise you are likely to get it again, by becoming re-infected!

Sexplained © 1995 Helen Knox

❖ be advised by the Doctor treating you

What about oral sex, anal sex and condoms?
❖ there is a risk of passing gonorrhoea by oral or anal sex
❖ see p.59 **'What *is* safer sex?'**

What complications can come from having gonorrhoea?
   men
❖ a tube inside the testicle(s) may become inflamed and swell (epidydimitis) - causing pain
❖ sterility of the affected testicle can occur (not enough fertile sperm to make a baby)
   women
❖ the fallopian tubes may become inflamed (salpingitis)
❖ you may get inflammation of the inside of the womb (endometritis) - although this can have other causes
❖ there may be an increased chance of tubal (ectopic) pregnancy
   both men and women
❖ there is an increased risk of infertility (being unable to have children)
❖ there may be 'septic arthritis of the joints'
❖ there may be skin boils
   babies may get
❖ 'sticky eye' and conjunctivitis (inflammation of the white area of the eye) if gonorrhoea is passed on from a Mother to her baby during vaginal delivery

How can I avoid getting gonorrhoea?
❖ take time to get to know your partner, although they may not own up to previous infections!
❖ see p.59 **'What *is* safer sex?'**

Sexplained © 1995 Helen Knox

Other name:
❖ inflammation of the liver

Where does it come from?
❖ the main viral causes are from:
  1 Hepatitis A virus
  2 Hepatitis B virus
  3 Hepatitis C virus
  4 Hepatitis D virus
  5 Hepatitis E virus
❖ other non-infectious causes of hepatitis are from the excess use of alcohol, some drugs and medication
❖ **this deals with causes 1-5 above, only**

How do I get hepatitis and what happens if I do?
the viruses are present in many things:

Hepatitis A - is generally found in:
❖ contaminated food or water supplies
❖ shellfish which are caught in contaminated waters
❖ areas of overcrowding and poor hygiene
❖ if infectious people are handling food in an unhygenic manner
❖ it is also present in human faeces (bowel waste) of infectious people
❖ it usually causes a short term illness

❖ a vaccination is available against 'hepatitis A' (this is a simple injection to help your body build immunity to the specific infection)
❖ for short term protection, one injection is available
❖ for longer term protection, a course of injections is available

Hepatitis B - also known as HBV (hepatitis B virus) - is found in:
❖ blood and body fluids - saliva, semen, vaginal secretions (sex), urine, sweat and tears of infected people
❖ contaminated drug injecting equipment, including needles & syringes, water ampoules (sealed glass capsules) or glasses, filters and spoons etc.
❖ some blood transfusions abroad

❖ it can lead to long term illness
❖ a vaccine is available against 'hepatitis B'

Hepatitis C - of which there are at least 6 types - each of those having many sub-types, is found in:
❖ contaminated blood in transfusions or shared drug injecting equipment, including needles, syringes, filters, spoons and water ampoules (sealed glass capsules) or glasses, as above
❖ it can be passed during sex
❖ this is considered more likely than was previously thought
❖ some blood transfusions abroad

❖ no vaccine is available for 'hepatitis C' yet, as there are so many different types and sub-types of the virus
❖ it can lead to long term illness

Sexplained © 1995 Helen Knox

Hepatitis D requires 'hepatitis B' to survive
* it is passed the same way
* vaccination against 'hepatitis B' will protect against 'hepatitis D'
* it can lead to long term illness

Hepatitis E - is found in contaminated drinking water - usually abroad - similar to 'hepatitis A'
* no vaccination is available yet

How long does it take to show in blood samples, if I catch it?
* Hepatitis A - 2 to 7 weeks
* Hepatitis B - 4 weeks to 6 months
* Hepatitis C - 5 to 12 weeks
* Hepatitis D - up to 6 month
* Hepatitis E - 4 to 8 weeks

Where can I get a blood test?
* your GP can arrange the blood test for you or you can go to a GUM/STD Clinic, where it is totally confidential
* if your GP is later asked to fill in insurance forms for you, there are often questions about sexually transmitted infections, which they have to answer
* the choice is yours

How infectious is hepatitis?
* 'hepatitis B and C' can be highly infectious, **much** more so than HIV / AIDS
* there are three different grades of 'infectiousness' for Hepatitis B, depending on the types of virus particles in the blood
  a) - **highly infectious** - you could pass the virus through unprotected sex (sex without a condom), sharing a toothbrush or razor, drug injecting equipment (as above) etc.
  b) - **mildly infectious** - you are less likely to pass the virus through unprotected sex (sex without a condom), but you cannot become a blood donor because your body (liver, kidneys etc.) has only partially cleared the virus
  c) - **not infectious** - your blood tests tell the Doctor that you have had 'hepatitis', but you have cleared the virus particles and cannot give the disease to anybody else

What might I notice?
* you may notice nothing at all! Many people don't even know they have hepatitis until they have a blood test to check
* you may notice general 'unwellness' (like 'flu')
* you may notice tiredness or fatigue
* your urine may be dark
* your bowel motions may be pale
* you may lose your appetite
* you may have abdominal tenderness and pain
* you may have a fever
* you may have night sweats
* you may itch and your skin may take on a 'yellow tinge' - indicating 'jaundice'
* the whites of your eyes may go yellow - indicating 'jaundice'

- ❖ you may have morning headaches
- ❖ you may go off smoking or alcohol

What tests would I have?

- ❖ specific blood tests to check which hepatitis virus you have
- ❖ if you become ill with hepatitis you may have liver function tests (special blood tests) and liver biopsy - taking a tiny sample of liver tissue, under local anaesthetic, which is sent to the laboratory to check the extent of any damage

If I have hepatitis, what treatment is there?

- ❖ the main treatment is rest, peace and quiet, so don't tire yourself out by trying to do too much, physically
- ❖ eat a healthy diet - with plenty of fresh produce
- ❖ avoid alcohol and other drugs, unless prescribed by the Doctor treating you
- ❖ some people benefit from aromatherapy and acupuncture to improve their general well-being
- ❖ you may be admitted to hospital
- ❖ if you have Hepatitis 'B' or 'C' you may be given a course of 'Interferon' injections
- ❖ your treatment depends upon how ill you are and which strain of the virus you have
- ❖ some people develop cirrhosis (pronounced 'si-ro-sis') of the liver (for which there are other causes)

What is cirrhosis of the liver?

- ❖ except from Hepatitis 'A', this is when blood is unable to flow freely through the liver and instead is diverted around it
- ❖ some people develop ascites, (pronounced 'a-site-eez') a swelling of the stomach (abdomen) with fluid, because the blood is unable to flow freely through the liver and does not contain enough protein
- ❖ ascites usually improves if salt is left out of the diet and the Doctor prescribes a 'diuretic' which will make the body pass out salt and water, through the kidneys, rather than the liver
- ❖ some people, with severe ascites, have to have their abdominal swelling 'drained' with a special instrument
- ❖ some people develop 'varices', (pronounced 'va-ri-seez') enlarged blood vessels around the stomach and lower end of the gullet (oesophagus)
- ❖ varices can cause bleeding from around the stomach because the diverted blood is under pressure and the blood vessels sometimes 'burst'
- ❖ this can be serious, even 'life threatening'
- ❖ lack of 'clotting factors' which are normally produced by the liver, can also make the problem worse (internal bleeding becomes more likely)
- ❖ cirrhosis cannot be 'treated' or 'cured' as such, by medical means, only its development

stopped
- any cirrhosis caused as a result of 'hepatitis' will remain even if the 'hepatitis' which caused it gets better
- some people with cirrhosis lead an entirely normal life
- other people with ascites or varices may need to have a liver transplant
- liver cancer may occur in people with long standing cirrhosis

What should I do after I finish the treatment?
- it depends upon how severely your liver has been damaged
- be guided by the Doctor treating you but you will probably be able to lead a perfectly normal lifestyle and simply have regular blood tests by your GP to monitor your health

What about my partner?
- be as open and honest as possible with other people for their protection
- they should be tested as soon as possible and if they are found not to have protection against the virus - they would be strongly advised to have the vaccination against 'hepatitis B' although if you have 'hepatitis C', there is no vaccine yet
- your partner may have other germs or a different 'strain' of the virus which might affect you
- if you find it hard to tell your partner - a Health Advisor at a GUM/STD clinic, or your Doctor, may be able to help you explain things more easily to them. They may feel angry or frightened, and have lots of questions

What about sex?
- be advised by the Doctor treating you
- you may decide on other forms of intimacy - rather than sex (see low risk activities and alternatives to sex in the section **'What *is* safer sex?'**)
- if you do have sex, condoms and extra lubricant are strongly advised
- **hepatitis is much easier to catch than HIV**
- see p.59 **'What *is* safer sex?'**

What about oral sex?
- 'hepatitis B and C' can be present in saliva if there are bleeding gums, cuts or sores in the mouth, or cut/chapped lips **(e.g. gums often bleed when newly brushed, so suck a mint before 'wet' kissing, to freshen your breath, instead)**
- it is important to protect yourself and your partner, even if you both have or have had the virus
- **'hepatitis A'** can pass by unprotected 'rimming' (anal licking)
- for oral sex to a man - the use of flavoured or non-spermicidal condoms is wise and they are designed for this
- for oral sex to a woman see p.59 **'What *is* safer sex?'** and its section on oral sex, on p.67

What about anal sex?
- this is 'high risk sex'
- hepatitis can pass this way
- condoms and extra lubricant should always be used
- see p.59 **'What *is* safer sex?'**

What about condoms?
- a correctly used condom - before ANY genital contact - can help to protect you from infection
- see p.59 **'What *is* safer sex?'**

What complications can come from having hepatitis?
- some people become chronic (long term - more than six months) carriers of the infection and many can pass the virus on for several years
- severe scarring of the liver can occur - leading to cirrhosis (see 'What is cirrhosis?')
- the blood supply in the liver may become blocked which can lead to one type of high blood pressure
- the immune system may be weakened
- some people become unable to tolerate alcohol
- some people develop cancer of the liver after having hepatitis
- some people become very ill and die from liver failure

How can I avoid getting hepatitis?
- have the vaccination
- take time to get to know your partner as well as they will let you!
- the careful and consistent use of condoms, even with another

method of birth control, is wise, as protection against infection

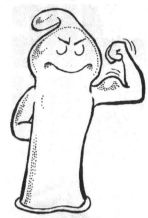

- don't share needles or injecting equipment, syringes, filters, water ampoules (sealed glass capsules) or glasses, spoons, etc.
- enjoy other forms of intimacy, rather than penetrative sex
- never assume that a clean looking person is clear of infection
- see p.59 **'What *is* safer sex?'**

Mother to baby infection
- if you are infected the baby can be vaccinated against 'hepatitis B' shortly after birth to prevent it getting the illness
- breast-feeding is good for the baby - but be advised by the Doctors treating you
- the baby remains 'at risk' if you have 'hepatitis C'

Some general points about hepatitis
- have the 'hepatitis B' vaccination as soon as possible if you are looking after someone with

hepatitis or if you feel you are 'at risk', then you know you have some protection, even if you make a mistake with the following general hygiene suggestions

❖ hepatitis is not caught by social contact i.e. shaking hands, hugging etc.

❖ the germs are passed in blood and blood stained body fluids - so, as long as you are careful with those, you minimise the risk of infection

❖ hepatitis can be a serious illness and is not one to be taken lightly

❖ you still have to be very careful if the person has 'hepatitis C' as there is no vaccination

❖ **'hepatitis B' virus can remain active in dried blood for over a week**

❖ **hepatitis is harder to destroy than HIV which dies in the air in a fairly short time**

❖ **take precautions and develop good habits of hygiene**

the vaccination

❖ see your Doctor within 36 hours if you feel you have been put 'at risk' of hepatitis B

❖ two injections can be given straight away (one a vaccine and the other 'antibodies') then the vaccination course continues - two more injections over 6 months for hepatitis B

if you *have* 'hepatitis'

❖ you do not need to have your own dishes and cutlery, as long as they are washed properly in **hot** soapy water, to kill the virus

❖ **but** in the early days of the illness it may be sensible to keep your own dishes and cutlery separate, so that no-one else can use them before they are washed

❖ **blood, urine and faeces** (bowel waste) are **highly infectious** and need extremely careful handling *(this includes handling babies nappies)*

cuts and spills

❖ cover **cuts or other open areas** (e.g. psoriasis or eczema skin conditions) with waterproof plaster before cleaning anything

❖ wear your own rubber gloves before dealing with infectious matter (don't let other people use the same gloves)

❖ wash your hands in soap and water after you finish and dry them on your own towel which no-one else should be allowed to use

❖ use disposable cloths to mop anything up - and dispose of them in a double wrapping of plastic

❖ use household bleach to disinfect and then dry any contaminated areas, with separate disposable cloths

❖ always wash hands, with soap and water, after using the 'loo'

women with hepatitis

❖ should dispose of sanitary towels carefully in double plastic wrapping, if throwing them out -

and then wash their hands with soap and water after doing so

❖ tampons can be flushed down the 'loo' as can some sanitary towels

if you get involved in <u>fights or with human bites</u>

❖ the infected blood should be mopped up, as above

❖ wounds on either party should be squeezed immediately, and made to bleed in order to clean out any infected matter as quickly as possible - then follow the normal procedures for wound care and see a Doctor

❖ either party should get the vaccination, if they are not already protected

<u>Other things to be careful about, where blood contamination can occur</u> : -

❖ don't share towels or nail files

❖ don't share toothbrushes, razors or blades with other people - gums may bleed - razors may cut skin - however careful you are

❖ don't share drug injecting equipment - needles, syringes, water ampoules (sealed glass capsules) or glasses, filters, spoons etc.

❖ **it is safer to suck a mint to freshen your breath when indulging in 'deep wet kissing' than to brush your teeth just before you have sex or kiss, as gums often bleed**

❖ always wash hands in soap and water after going to the toilet

❖ acupuncture - check that the therapist uses disposable needles or sterilizes them properly between clients

❖ electrolysis - as above

❖ body piercing or 'stone insertion' - as above

❖ tattooing - as above - but also ensure that the ink has not been used with a previous customer as this could risk 'pooling' the virus and passing it on via the ink

❖ inform your Dentist if you have, or have had, hepatitis - even though they would be using 'universal precautions' and treating everyone the same. If you don't tell them there could be extra problems stopping any bleeding if your liver is affected at the time

❖ contact sports - see 'fights or human bites'

❖ inform anyone else who needs to know

<u>your local council</u>

❖ hepatitis is a 'notifiable disease' - so the Environmental Health Department of your local council may contact you to ensure safe disposal of infectious material e.g. soiled dressings, heavily soiled bedding (if you are unable to 'hot-wash' them thoroughly in a washing machine) or incontinence sheets, anything you have used to mop up any spillages of blood, vomit, faeces etc. and any other infected matter which is being thrown out. They should be kept separately in special containers before being collected for incineration (to be burnt)

the test

* whether you have the 'hepatitis test' from your GP or at a GUM/STD clinic is up to you
* a GUM/STD clinic, is confidential your GP may later have to fill in insurance forms for you which can have questions about infections on them - they have to answer these
* your GP is not informed of your attendance at a GUM/STD clinic, unless you give your permission for them to do so

Note:

* *in the tiny amount of blood involved in a 'needle stick injury' (syringe stab) the chance of getting HIV (if it is present), is 0.3% but the chance of getting hepatitis (if it is present) is 30% = 100 times more likely*
* **many people are 'hepatitis positive' and do not realise**
* *over half of the tested injecting (intravenous) drug users in the UK are positive to 'hepatitis C' - for which there is no vaccine*
* **no-one can tell by looking at another person who is infectious or what they may have, so do look after yourself and don't risk your life**
* **it depends upon the state of both your mouths and whether there is blood in the saliva - a tiny amount is sufficient, to pass on hepatitis or herpes** see p.59 'What *is* safer sex?'

Other name:
❖ cold sores

Where does it come from?
There are several different types of herpes virus including:-
1 - herpes zoster - also known as shingles
2 - herpes simplex virus 1 (HSV 1)
3 - herpes simplex virus 2 (HSV 2)
4 - cytomegalovirus (CMV)
5 - Epstein-Barr virus infection - which causes glandular fever.
6 - human herpes virus 6

There are two types of herpes simplex virus.
❖ HSV 1 **usually** causes 'cold sores' around the mouth and nose, but can affect the genitalia ('down below')
❖ HSV 2 **usually** causes sores in the genital and anal areas, but can affect the mouth

How do I get herpes?
❖ it is transmitted by sexual or close physical contact - when the sores are open (wet)
❖ genital herpes can pass to the mouth if oral sex is practiced - and oral herpes can pass to the genital area ('down below')
❖ oral herpes can pass by kissing when sores are wet (this also applies to children kissing each other)

How long does it take to show?
❖ usually 3 - 6 days for the first attack

recurrent attacks: 1 - 2 days after something sets it off again
❖ the recurrent cause may not always be recognised

What might I notice?
for men and women
❖ herpes can be a recurrent infection, with the first attack being the most painful
❖ many little 'blisters' & 'ulcers' appear anywhere 'down below'
❖ they start off small, clear or yellowy
❖ then may join together forming larger sore areas, up to about 2 cms across
❖ recurrent attacks usually occur at the same site as the first attack
❖ you may feel generally unwell, with the first attack in particular
❖ women may retain urine from fear of the pain felt when passing it
❖ there may be tingling or pain in the lower back, buttocks or back of the leg before an attack
❖ there may be an offensive vaginal discharge and soreness
❖ there may be soreness or irritation 'down below' and/or in the 'back passage'
❖ this may lead to bowel retention and constipation
❖ the herpes virus stays in the body for life
❖ recurrent attacks usually occur less frequently, as time goes by

What tests would I have?
❖ visual diagnosis by an experienced Doctor
❖ laboratory tests - blood tests and

Sexplained © 1995 Helen Knox

swabs taken of the discharge

What treatment is there, if I have herpes?

❖ salt baths
❖ the usual treatment, for the first or severe attacks, is a medication called Acyclovir (or Zovirax) in tablet form

What should I do after I finish the treatment?

❖ it may take 2 - 3 weeks for the initial sores to heal up
❖ it is not necessary to return to the clinic for recurrent attacks, but you are welcome to do so, if you wish

What about my partner?

❖ it is sensible to be open and tell your partner about it
❖ they will have questions and fears which you or a Health Advisor can help them overcome
❖ they can always talk to your Health Advisor who will explain the infection to them, if you can't

What about sex?

❖ this must be avoided until all the sores have healed up
❖ this is because the virus can easily be spread whilst the sores are 'wet'

What about oral sex, anal sex and condoms?

❖ 'cold sores' are oral herpes and can pass to the genital area ('down below') when 'wet' and genital herpes can pass to the

mouth when 'wet' so avoid contact at those times
❖ when they have dried up you are relatively safe to have sex again
❖ see p.59 **'What *is* safer sex?'**

What complications can come from having herpes?
in pregnancy

❖ if you have the first attack of genital herpes during early pregnancy, there is a risk to the baby
❖ many doctors advise a 'caesarean' delivery of the baby if the first attack occurs in the last few weeks of the pregnancy or if there is a recurrent attack on the day of delivery, or immediately before it

General possible complications of herpes:
there may be one or more of the following:

❖ severe burning or stabbing pain along a nerve line (neuralgia)
❖ inflammation of the root of a nerve (radiculitis)
❖ constipation - from fear of the pain involved in opening the back passage (anus)
❖ anxiety
❖ depression
❖ 'impotence' or inability to get and keep an erection - from the fear of pain or of passing on the infection
❖ strain on relationships
❖ fear of cervical cancer (as genital herpes was previously believed to be a risk factor for cervical cancer)

How can I avoid getting herpes?

❖ never assume that a 'clean looking' person is clear of infection

❖ don't have sex with someone when they have open (wet) sores

❖ be careful, or don't kiss people with open (wet) 'cold sores' on their mouth or have oral sex with them at that time

❖ talk to a Health Advisor if you want further advice

❖ see p.59 **'What *is* safer sex?'**

Other name:
- ❖ human immunodeficiency virus

Where does it come from?
- ❖ it is a virus which lives off its host and multiplies within it
- ❖ HIV attaches itself to the white blood cells, which normally help us fight off infections
- ❖ there are two strains of the virus - HIV1 & HIV2

How is it passed on?
it is passed by the exchange of blood or other body fluids from one infected person to another person for example, by-
- ❖ unprotected penetrative vaginal or anal sex
- ❖ oral sex, if cuts or sores are present
- ❖ sharing any equipment used for injecting drugs - needles, syringes, glasses or water ampoules (sealed glass capsules), filters, spoons etc.
- ❖ blood transfusions or organ transplant - although in the UK and 'western world' they are all tested for HIV before use
- ❖ infected breast milk
- ❖ from mother to baby in pregnancy, where there is a 12-30% risk of passing HIV to the baby

How long does it take to show?
- ❖ from the anticipated time of infection, it takes three to six months for most people to react enough for the laboratory to detect an 'antibody reaction' to HIV in their blood

What might I notice?
- ❖ there are usually no specific signs or symptoms to tell that you have contracted HIV

What tests would I have?
- ❖ a specific blood test is necessary at present
- ❖ this only tells your 'HIV status' (if you were HIV antibody positive or negative) three months ago, not for example, yesterday
- ❖ you may be asked to wait three months to have the test, or if you are given the test straight away, advised to have it repeated in three months. Either have 'no sex' or only 'protected' sex in that time and you will be advised not to put yourself at further risk

What treatment is there, if I have HIV?
- ❖ if you **know** you are 'HIV antibody positive' (have caught the virus) and you get common illnesses, your Doctor will probably give you antibiotics, or other medicine, to keep you healthy and well
- ❖ if they don't know you're HIV positive they might not give you antibiotics
- ❖ the reason for this is that normally, the 'immune system' fights off infection with only minimal help - but if you are 'HIV antibody positive', you could have reduced resistance and ability to fight off infection
- ❖ the aim is to keep you healthy for

longer and delay the onset of AIDS

❖ at this time, scientists are working hard to find a cure

What should I do after I finish the treatment?

❖ be advised by the Doctor treating you

❖ regular medical 'check-ups' are sensible

❖ hospital clinics can refer you to all the other departments of the hospital for care, including dental care, if you find it difficult to get this help elsewhere

What about my partner(s)?

❖ your partner should be checked in case they have the infection or to keep safe if they don't

❖ telling them may be hard for you and something you may not feel able to do immediately

❖ discuss this with your Health Advisor as they have experience of the dilemma of 'who to tell, when and why'

What about sex?

❖ the consistent use of condoms is strongly advised

❖ you may prefer to enjoy other forms of intimacy rather than penetrative sex

❖ see *'low risk activities and alternatives to penetrative sex'* in the section **'What *is* safer sex?'** p.59

What about oral sex, anal sex and condoms?

❖ it is important to protect yourself and your partner, even if you are both HIV antibody positive

❖ they may have other germs or a different strain of HIV which might affect you and make you more ill, if you catch them

❖ see p.59 **'What *is* safer sex?'**

What complications can come from having it?

❖ HIV can lead to AIDS

❖ you could be perfectly healthy for about ten years without even realising you have been infected

❖ during that time you could infect other people

In short - HIV is caught - the person may not feel any different for many years - then they may have difficulty fighting off minor illnesses. This weakens their immune system. With a little more time, the immune system

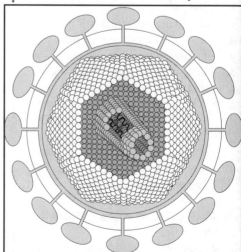

Sexplained © 1995 Helen Knox

cannot fight off invading germs and AIDS starts to take over. AIDS can make you vulnerable to illnesses which the body can no longer fight off and destroy

Should I be tested for HIV?

❖ the choice has to be yours and you should not decide to have the test without realising its implications

❖ the 'Health Advisors', in GUM/STD clinics, would explain these to you **before** you are tested and help you assess your own situation

❖ you should be open and honest with them though, for it helps them work out your 'risk status'

❖ there are **advantages** to having the test, although you may not want to know, or are too scared to know - you could be worrying for no reason, and the only way to put your mind at ease is to be tested

❖ the **disadvantages** are more to do with insurance companies, mortgage requests etc., although their attitude and the associated 'stigma' is changing

❖ you can discuss it thoroughly with a 'Health Advisor' at a GUM/STD clinic

❖ if in doubt about anything - ask questions and keep asking until you have your answers

Will my Doctor suggest I have the test?

❖ generally, it is left up to you to decide about this

❖ they may ask you to have it, if you are ill and they cannot find out what is wrong with you otherwise sometimes people who are 'HIV antibody positive' have a lower resistance to sexually transmitted infections than other people - so, if you keep getting recurrences of infection, it **may** be suggested

❖ they would only ask this of you, after trying the usual treatments without success

How can I avoid getting HIV?

❖ take time to get to know your partner before having penetrative sex together

❖ careful and consistent use of condoms - even with another method of birth control - is wise, as protection against infection

❖ don't share needles or injecting equipment of any sort if you use drugs

❖ you may decide on other forms of intimacy, rather than penetrative sex **(see low risk activities in 'What is safer sex?' section p. 60)**

❖ never assume that a 'clean looking person' is clear of infection

❖ see p.59 **'What is safer sex?'**

❖ protect yourself - **use condoms every time you have sex**

There are many leaflets and books written about AIDS and HIV which explain the infection in greater detail

❖ perhaps, you may like to make a list of questions you want answered, before you speak to the 'health professionals' they won't mind

Other names:
- ❖ pubic lice or 'crabs'
- ❖ head lice
- ❖ body lice

What are they?
- ❖ they are tiny parasites or creatures

How do I get them?
- ❖ close body contact - they can be sexually transmitted, but not always

How long do they take to show?
- ❖ it may be immediate - after the adult louse bites you, to feed
- ❖ it is often noticed in 1 - 2 weeks
- ❖ once they arrive, pubic lice and head lice live on the body at all times and crawl to all hairy areas of the body
- ❖ body lice live in seams of clothing and crawl onto the body to feed
- ❖ the adults mate and after 48 hours the female lays her eggs (nits) at the base of hairs, the 'nit' sticks to the hair - and as this grows, the 'nit' moves with it, away from the skin
- ❖ the 'nits' hatch after a week and travel back towards the skin for another week until they mature into an adult louse or 'crab'
- ❖ each 'crab' (adult louse) lives about a month, during which time it can lay about 50 eggs!

What might I notice?
- ❖ you will probably itch
- ❖ you may notice 'little creatures' crawling about in your hair

- ❖ you may notice small dark spots from where they inject their saliva whilst feeding
- ❖ scratching may cause the skin to bleed and crust over - some sore areas may become infected

What tests would I have?
- ❖ the Doctor will examine you
- ❖ samples of the lice may be viewed under a microscope

What treatment is there if I have pubic lice?
- ❖ the treatment is the same as for 'scabies' (see 'scabies') but repeated after a week - this gives time for any unhatched 'nits' to hatch and then be killed by the treatment

What should I do after I finish the treatment?
- ❖ the Doctor may want to see you again to be sure they have all gone

What about my partner?
- ❖ they, and all people you are in close conttact with, should be seen and treated

What about sex?
- ❖ this should be avoided until you are clear of lice to avoid re-infestation

What about oral sex, anal sex and condoms?
- ❖ see p.59 **'What *is* safer sex?'**

How can I avoid getting them?

❖ avoid close contact with people
who have them and don't share
bedding, towels or underwear etc.

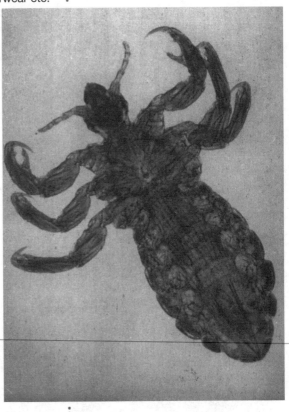

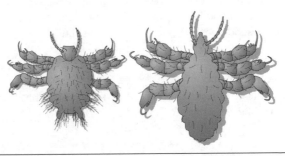

Pediculosis pubis
(pubic louse)

Pediculosis corporis
(body louse)

Sexplained © 1995 Helen Knox

Other name:
❖ 'NSU'

Where does it come from?
❖ several germs may cause NSU but the most common one is called 'chlamydia' (pronounced 'cla-mi-dea')
❖ other causes can be trichomonas (TV / 'trich')
❖ or 'thrush'
❖ it may be secondary to other infections in the urine passage
❖ it may come from having or performing unprotected oral sex with a sore throat or other mouth infection

How do I get NSU?
❖ it is usually sexually transmitted

How long does it take to show?
❖ some people don't notice anything at all
❖ it usually takes 2 - 4 weeks but symptoms may show within a few days from the time of contact
❖ or if it is mild, it may not be noticed for several months

What might I notice?
men
❖ you would probably notice a discharge from your penis
❖ this may be only a little and milky in appearance, although sometimes it can be as much as with gonorrhoea
❖ there may be a 'burning' sensation or general discomfort when you pass urine
❖ this may be particularly noticeable first thing in the morning
❖ there may be general discomfort of the penis
❖ there may be 'wetness' or 'dribbling' after passing urine
❖ ejaculation may be painful
❖ you may have difficulty maintaining an erection
❖ some men notice sore testicles
❖ you may not notice anything at all!
women
❖ usually there is very little to notice in women
❖ examination may also reveal very little
❖ there may be inflammation of the fallopian tubes (salpingitis) which suggests you have an infection
❖ sex may become painful
❖ pelvic pain may become prolonged if you are not treated
❖ this may lead to 'infertility' (being unable to have a baby)

What tests would I have?
❖ ***men*** will have urine tests, so try not to pass urine for at least 4 hours before giving a sample
❖ ***men and women*** will have swabs taken (when a special cotton wool bud is wiped through the discharge) and checked in the laboratory

What treatment is there, if I have NSU?
❖ antibiotics

What should I do after I finish the treatment?
❖ you will probably be asked to

return to the clinic which treated you, for a check-up

* this is to ensure that the infection has all gone and that you don't have anything else
* some women notice that 'thrush' can start-up after certain antibiotics are taken and they then need treatment for that, too

What about my partner?

* they must be checked at a GUM/STD clinic
* they may not complain of anything but may have an infection
* if they are not treated too, there is a risk of you becoming re-infected by them
* even if no infection is found in them, they will be given the same treatment as you 'just in case' - as NSU can be difficult to diagnose in women

What about sex?

* this should be avoided, even with a condom, until the treatment is finished and you are given the 'all clear' by the Doctor treating you

What about oral sex, anal sex and condoms?

* NSU can pass by oral or penetrative sex
* see p.59 **'What *is* safer sex?'**

What complications can come from having NSU?

if treated quickly there are not usually complications but occasionally it can lead to:

men
* the prostate gland becoming inflamed (prostatitis)
* the testicles becoming tender and a Doctor should see them

women
* the fallopian tubes can become inflamed, which may lead to pelvic inflammatory disease (see 'PID')
* inflammation of the glands at the entrance to the vagina (Bartholinitis)
* sex may be painful
* pelvic pain may continue long term
* 'infertility' could be a result (being unable to have a baby)

How can I avoid getting NSU?

* take time to get to know your partner
* see p.59 **'What *is* safer sex?'**

(for women only)

Other names:
* P.I.D. or pelvic infection

What is it?
* inflammation inside the lower abdominal area (tubes, uterus or womb)

Where does PID come from?
* usually a germ (or bacterium) such as chlamydia, gonorrhoea, gardnerella and ureoplasma hominis, to name but a few

How do I get PID?
* it is sexually transmitted
* it can lie 'dormant' (sleeping) for a long time, then lead to P.I.D.

How long does it take to show?
* it depends on the infection - from days to months

What might I notice?
suddenly : acutely : immediately - you may notice one or more of the following:-
* low abdominal pain
* pain during sex (dyspareunia)
* back pain
* high temperature (38∞ C) and shivering (feeling hot and cold)
* unusual vaginal discharge - which may be thick, or thin and 'smelly'
* occasionally irregular bleeding
* heavy bleeding
* or spotting between periods
longer term -
* pelvic pain, either 'on and off' or constantly - this may be centrally,

or to one or both sides
* pelvic pain during sex
* low back pain
* feeling generally unwell
* painful periods
* reduced fertility
* passing urine more often
* pain on passing urine
* pelvic pain during periods
* pelvic pain during ovulation

What tests would I have?
* a 'swab' or sample of the discharge is taken by wiping a special cotton wool bud through the discharge, which is then sent to the laboratory
* internal examination by a Doctor if it is persistent, an ultrasound may be undertaken
* and perhaps laparoscopy - when a Doctor looks inside the abdomen with a special telescope
* *NOTE* - the Doctor needs to 'rule out' other possible causes of pelvic pain - e.g. adhesions or 'stickiness' inside, endometriosis (when the tissue lining the womb is present at other areas of the pelvic cavity), problems with the ovaries, fibroids (muscular growths of the uterus/womb which are non-cancerous), ectopic (tubal) pregnancy, acute appendicitis, irritable bowel syndrome, and pelvic congestion

What treatment is there, if I have PID?
* antibiotics - which must all be taken correctly
* NO ALCOHOL should be

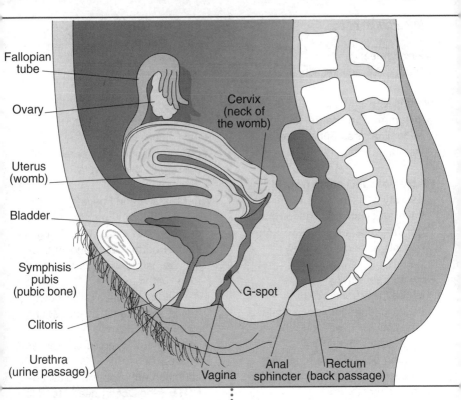

Fallopian tube

Ovary

Uterus (womb)

Bladder

Symphisis pubis (pubic bone)

Clitoris

Urethra (urine passage)

Cervix (neck of the womb)

G-spot

Vagina

Anal sphincter

Rectum (back passage)

consumed whilst taking them

❖ P.I.D. can recur more readily if it is not eliminated at the start

❖ in some cases, surgery is required

❖ sometimes hospital admission is necessary

What about my partner?

❖ **they must be checked** thoroughly at a GUM/STD clinic and **treated** for any infections **as soon as possible**

❖ they don't always cause problems beforehand but some of the germs can cause infertility in **men** treatment is **essential** to prevent re-infection

What about sex?

❖ it is sensible not to have sex with anyone until you have been advised that it is safe to resume - and until your partner has been cleared of infection, too

❖ otherwise you are likely to become re-infected

What about oral sex, anal sex and condoms?

❖ see p.59 **'What *is* safer sex?'**

What complications can come from having PID?

❖ left untreated, acute P.I.D. could become chronic (long term)

❖ there is a much higher risk of

❖ future tubal (ectopic) pregnancy
❖ there is a risk of further attacks
❖ there is a greater chance of 'infertility' (being unable to have a baby) due to tubal damage

How can I avoid getting PID?
❖ the careful and consistent use of condoms - even with another method of birth control, is wise - as protection against infection
❖ reduce casual sex/number of partners
❖ if any infections are caught, prompt, correct diagnosis and treatment is essential
❖ have regular check-ups at a GUM/STD clinic if you are concerned
❖ see p.59 **'What *is* safer sex?'**

Where do they come from?

❖ they are 'mites' called 'sarcoptes scabiei'

How do I get them?

❖ by close physical contact

How long do they take to show?

❖ first attack - 3 to 6 weeks after infection
❖ it takes 3 to 4 days from the time the female lays her eggs until they 'hatch'
❖ after 'hatching' - the larvae migrate to a skin fold and moult several times
❖ they take about two weeks to mature

What might I notice?

❖ there is usually itching which is worse at night when you are warm
❖ small raised spots and 'burrows'
(like raised, red, scratch lines) appear - usually on the genitalia ('down below') hands, forearms, between the fingers, at the wrists, buttocks, around the nipples in women & under arms etc.
❖ a rash

What tests would I have?

❖ visually, as they are usually easily recognised
❖ this is confirmed by scraping the burrows and examination of these samples under a microscope

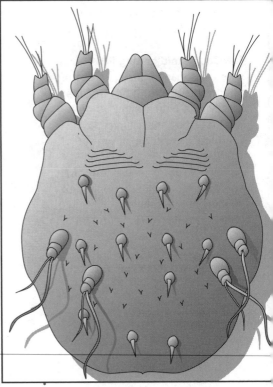

What treatment is there, if I have scabies?

❖ there are lotions to kill the 'mites'
❖ clothing, bed linen and towels should all be changed and washed thoroughly

❖ **Note**: the symptoms may take a week or two to clear, so do not repeat the treatment frequently, otherwise dermatitis (skin inflammation) may occur

What should I do after I finish the treatment?

❖ be guided by the Doctor treating you

❖ they will probably ask you to return, (perhaps more than once) to ensure that all the scabies have gone

What about my partner?

❖ he/she should be seen and treated, too - as should all family members or residents of the same accommodation, if they have symptoms

What about sex?

❖ this should be avoided until you and your partner are clear of scabies to avoid re-infestation

What about oral sex, anal sex and condoms?

❖ as this involves close physical contact, avoid sexual contact until after the scabies have cleared, to avoid re-infestation

❖ see p.59 **'What *is* safer sex?'**

How can I avoid getting scabies?

❖ try and avoid close physical contact with people you know to have it - until they are treated

❖ don't share towels, bedding, underwear or clothing with other people

'Norwegian' scabies (a different variety) ***may occur in:***

❖ overcrowded institutions with poor sanitary conditions

❖ people on certain medication which suppresses their immune system

Sexplained © 1995 Helen Knox

Other name:
* 'the pox'

Where does it come from?
* it is caused by a spiral shaped germ called 'treponema pallidum'

How do I get syphilis?
* it is sexually transmitted

How long does syphilis take to show?
* usually 14 - 35 days (2-5 weeks) after contact. It could be from 10 - 90 days (1 week - 3 months)

What might I notice?
*_men and women_*
The FIRST stage
* is usually the appearance of a small red spot, which loses its surface area, leaving an ulcer
* this is usually round and painless, with a clean surface
* left untreated, this ulcer is likely to grow to about 2cms and then slowly start to heal itself, in four to eight weeks
* there is unlikely to be a scar
* the surrounding area is likely to be swollen
* there may be enlargement of the glands in the groin and other areas

The SECOND stage
* is usually 6 - 8 weeks after infection
* there is usually a skin rash on the body - in particular palms of the hands, soles of the feet and on the chest/trunk
* moist areas of the body may be ulcerated
* various glands may enlarge and feel tender
* rarely, hair may fall out
* hepatitis (liver inflammation) may occur

The THIRD stage
* usually 3 to 30 years after untreated infection!
* it affects the brain, to cause 'general paralysis of the nervous system' (or when the brain is so damaged by syphilis that there is serious nerve damage, causing paralysis all over the body)
* blindness and visual problems
* heart and bone changes
* there may be gradual destruction of the bones and flesh

*_mother to baby_*
* the baby is vulnerable to infection by syphilis after the 16th week of pregnancy - so good ante-natal care is vital
* *in the UK all ante-natal patients have a blood test for syphilis*
* if it is diagnosed the woman can be treated and the baby protected
* *left untreated, the baby could be deformed or die*

What tests would I have?
* swabs and blood tests

What treatment is there, if I have syphilis?
* antibiotics

What should I do after I finish the treatment?

❖ you will be asked to return to the clinic treating you and have the tests repeated, to check that the infection has cleared

What about my partner?

❖ it is essential that your partner is checked for syphilis and treated if they have it

What about sex?

❖ this should be avoided until your treatment - and that of your partner - has been completed and you are told it is safe to have sex again by the Doctor treating you

❖ otherwise you risk becoming re-infected

What about oral sex, anal sex and condoms?

❖ syphilis can pass by oral or penetrative sex

❖ see p.59 **'What *is* safer sex?'**

What complications can come from having syphilis?

❖ see Stage 1, Stage 2 and Stage 3 above

How can I avoid getting syphilis?

❖ take time to get to know your partner

❖ the careful and consistent use of condoms, even with another method of birth control - is wise, as protection against infection

❖ careful partner selection - reduce casual sex / the number of partners

❖ never assume that a 'clean looking' person is clear of infection

❖ see p.59 **'What *is* safer sex?'**

IF LEFT UNTREATED, SYPHILIS CAN KILL!

Sexplained © 1995 Helen Knox

Other names:
- candidiasis, candida albicans or monilia infection

Where does it come from?
- it is a yeast which lives within all of us
- this is not necessarily a sexually transmitted infection, although it can be

What can make it show up in me?
'thrush' (or the yeast which lives in all of us), usually causes no problems and we don't even notice it is there but it can 'flare up' when the normal conditions in the vagina (or other moist areas of the body) are altered
this can be :-
- in pregnancy
- with diabetes
- after antibiotics, which can alter the usual balance of conditions in the vagina
- with some types of anaemia

What might I notice?
women may notice
- vulval and vaginal irritation (itchiness 'down below')
- pain on passing urine
- white vaginal discharge (like cottage cheese)
men may notice
- irritation of the 'glans' (knob/helmet of the penis) and 'prepuce' (foreskin)
- uncircumcised men are more susceptible and the foreskin may swell, tighten and require circumcision (surgical removal)

What tests would I have?
- swabs would be taken and sent to the laboratory to confirm the diagnosis
- your urine may be tested for 'glucose'/sugar to exclude diabetes

What treatment is there if I have thrush?
medical treatment
for both men and women -
- creams: twice daily for 14 days
or for women
- pessaries - vaginal tablets
- capsule - single oral dose
- **all the treatments should be taken as advised by the Doctor to ensure best results**

complimentary treatment for women -
- live natural yoghurt inserted vaginally via a tampon should help restore the 'normal' conditions in the vagina
- a very weak solution of vinegar inserted vaginally via a tampon or in a bath
- this, too, helps to re-balance the conditions in the vagina
- good personal hygiene
- bathe your 'private area' regularly with running water
- wash from front to back, to prevent bowel germs being easily transferred to the vagina and urine passage (which may lead to infection), then dry gently with a towel - 'dab', don't rub or scratch the sore areas
- alternatively dry the area with a

cool hairdryer, very carefully

❖ some people find that changing their diet to one with less yeast and sugar is very helpful

❖ ask your Doctor for advice

What should I do after I finish the treatment?

❖ follow the suggestions below about how to avoid getting thrush

What about my partner?

❖ your partner should be checked at a GUM/STD clinic they have symptoms

❖ if they are left untreated there is a risk that *your* thrush will return

What about sex?

❖ sex should be avoided whilst you are having treatment

What about oral sex, anal sex and condoms?

❖ thrush can pass by oral or penetrative sex

❖ see p.59 **'What *is* safer sex?'**

How can I avoid getting thrush?

❖ avoid tights or tight trousers

❖ don't use strongly scented soaps, bubble baths or disinfectants in the bath

❖ avoid vaginal deodorants

❖ some women prefer to use sanitary towels instead of tampons when having a 'period'

❖ wear cotton underwear rather than nylon or synthetic underwear

❖ practice good personal hygiene

❖ always wipe from 'front to back' after going to the toilet

❖ avoid sex if you have symptoms

❖ make sure that your partner is treated or you may easily get get re-infected!

❖ it is not recommended to have sex whilst being treated, even with a condom - the creams may affect the rubber of the condom which may then fail/break/burst! The friction involved may damage the sore vaginal surface. This may cause more pain and take longer to heal.

❖ try to ensure good general health - i.e. good diet with plenty of fluids, enough sleep and try to avoid emotional upsets

❖ **Lastly - do not assume you have 'thrush' - go for a proper check up at a GUM/ STD clinic**

(pronounced 'tri-ko-monas')

Other names:
❖ T.V. , 'trich'

Where does it come from?
❖ it is a parasite called 'trachomonas vaginalis'

How do I get TV?
❖ it is sexually transmitted

How long does it take to show?
❖ usually 1 - 2 weeks, although it may lie dormant ('sleeping')

What might I notice?
you may notice one or more of the following:-
women
❖ there is usually an increased vaginal discharge which is yellow, frothy and smelly
❖ soreness of the vagina and vulva (private area)
❖ burning pain when passing urine
❖ uncomfortable sex
men
❖ usually have no signs or symptoms
❖ occasionally there may be pain when passing urine
❖ there may be a discharge from the penis
❖ it often presents as NSU (see NSU)

What tests would I have?
❖ a swab (or sample taken by wiping a special cotton wool bud through the discharge) would be taken and viewed under a microscope
❖ you would also be given a full STD screen (check-up)

What treatment is there, if I have TV?
❖ antibiotics
❖ it is important **not** to consume **alcohol** whilst taking these tablets, as they react together and may make you feel sick

What should I do after I finish the treatment?
❖ be advised by the Doctor or clinic treating you - especially if you have any other infection as well - they may want to see you again
❖ it is wise to be checked again at a GUM/STD clinic after treatment, to be sure it has all gone

What about my partner?
❖ they should be seen in a GUM/STD clinic and checked thoroughly
❖ trichomonas can be difficult to find in men - even if a female partner has symptoms

What about sex?
❖ this should be avoided until your treatment - and that of your partner - has been completed,
❖ otherwise you may become re-infected!

What about oral sex, anal sex and condoms?
❖ TV can pass by oral or penetrative sex

❖ see p.59 **'What *is* safer sex?'**

What complications can come from having TV?

❖ in rare cases the infection can come back even though both partners have been treated
❖ if this happens to you a longer course of treatment is necessary

How can I avoid getting TV?

❖ take time to get to know your partner
❖ never assume that a 'clean looking' person is clear of infection
❖ see p.59 **'What *is* safer sex?'**

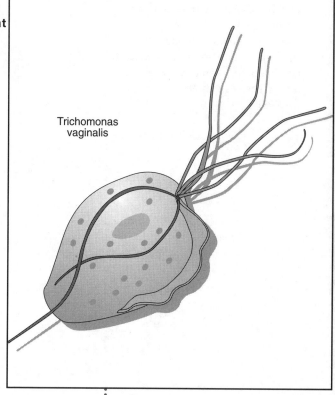

Trichomonas vaginalis

Sexplained © 1995 Helen Knox

(TSS)

- ❖ tampons left inside the vagina for a long time - or forgotten - may influence changes in the normal vaginal conditions and cause problems
- ❖ if this is in the presence of the bacteria or germ called 'staphylococcus' TSS can occur
- ❖ TSS can cause 'septicaemia' (blood poisoning) which is **a life threatening condition,** and has to be treated with antibiotics
- ❖ the use of sanitary towels rather than tampons on 'light flow' days may be helpful and does not carry the same risk
- ❖ many women have changed from using tampons (internal sanitary protection) to sanitary towels to avoid the risk of 'toxic shock syndrome'

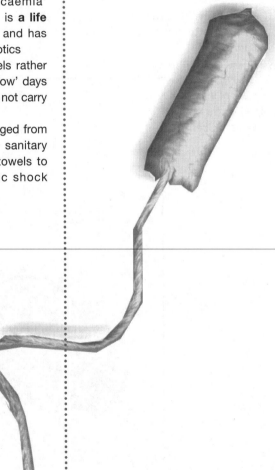

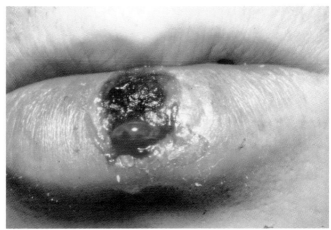

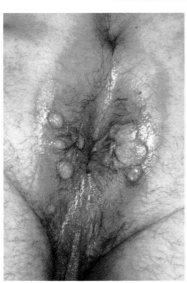

Top: SYPHILIS – on a lip (*not* to be confused with Herpes or cigarette burn!)

Left: SECONDARY SYPHILIS RASH around anal area

Below: SECONDARY SYPHILIS RASH

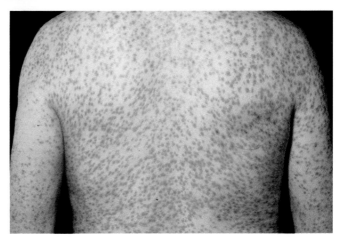

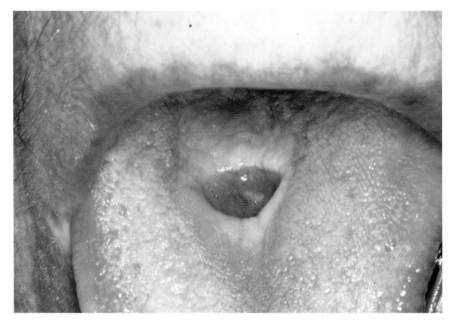

SYPHILIS – hole forming in a tongue

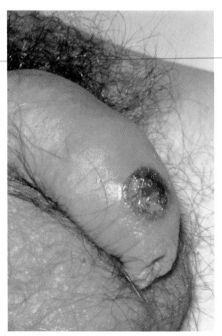

SYPHILIS – first stage

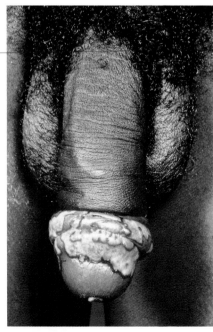

BALANITIS

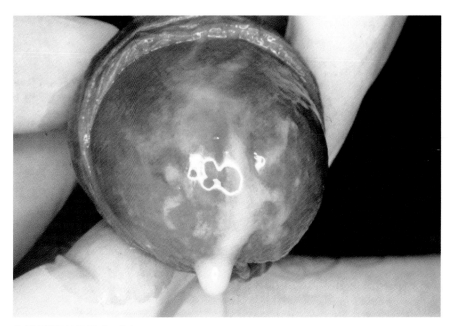

GONORRHOEA (male)
(Photo courtesy of Dr. K. C. Mohanty)

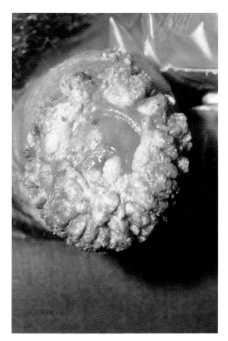

GENITAL WARTS (male)
(Photo courtesy of Dr. K. C. Mohanty)

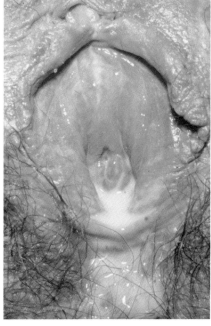

TRICHOMONIASIS VAGINALIS (T.V.)

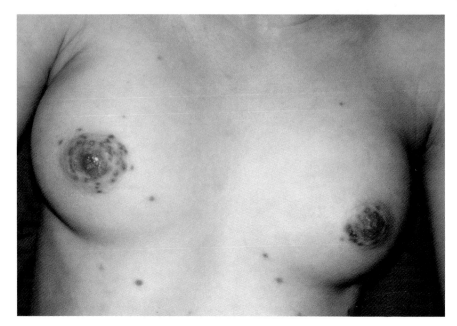

HERPES – around a woman's nipples

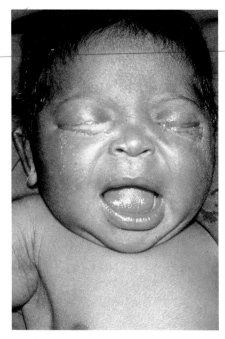

GONORRHOEA – caught from infected
mother during vaginal delivery

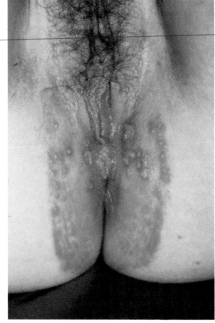

HERPES GENITALIS

❖ It is sensible for all men and women to be 'breast aware'

❖ to know the look, shape and texture of your breasts and to check them on a regular basis, after a period

❖ breast cancer affects one woman in twelve

❖ it is rare in men, but not unknown

❖ nine out of ten lumps which are found are not malignant (cancerous) - so if you find a lump, act quickly and let a Doctor check it

❖ you can either visit your GP or go to a Family Planning / Well Woman Clinic

❖ in the UK, women aged 50 to 65 are automatically invited for free 'mammography' (special breast X-ray) on a three yearly basis

What should I look for when I check my breasts?

❖ you are looking for **any** changes to the usual look or feel of your breast

❖ watch for any change to the nipple(s) and any discharge or secretion from them

❖ watch for any change in the direction the nipple(s) point, and any puckering or swelling of the skin

❖ any bulges in the breast contour need checking, as do the appearance of 'orange peel' skin, dimpling or tethering. (i.e. as if something is stuck to the inside of the breast, holding the skin back)

❖ swelling of the upper arm or armpit should arouse your suspicion and be checked

first:

❖ look at yourself in the mirror - standing upright - then leaning forwards - then tilting sideways - with your arms by your sides

❖ put your hands on your head (to stretch the breast tissue) and repeat looking, moving and checking as above, still looking in the mirror

❖ place your hands on your hips and repeat viewing, moving and checking again, as above

secondly:

❖ in a bath or lying on the bed (wherever you are most comfortable) - with one arm stretched behind your head, feel the opposite breast in a firm but gentle manner, with the flat of your hand

❖ start by squeezing the nipple and look for any fluid coming out

❖ feel, with your hand, in a 'Catherine wheel' motion around the nipple area, round and round the breast area and up into the armpit area

❖ all this time, be aware of the lumps you are feeling

❖ you will find lumps the first time you check, as the breasts are made up of many glands, surrounded by fat

❖ these lumps and bumps form a 'base line' from which you can notice any changes

❖ be comfortable and relaxed whilst checking

❖ when you make 'breast awareness' part of your routine health care, the stress of regular checking gets less

❖ if you are ever in doubt - ask your Doctor or Family Planning / Well Woman Clinic to check them for you

Sexplained © 1995 Helen Knox

- **MEN** should check themselves, too the same technique applies
- partners can check each others breasts

- other techniques may be suggested but the aim is to check the vulnerable areas

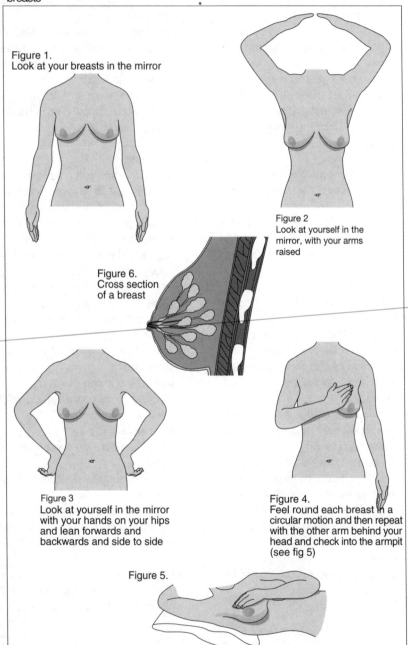

Figure 1.
Look at your breasts in the mirror

Figure 2
Look at yourself in the mirror, with your arms raised

Figure 6.
Cross section of a breast

Figure 3
Look at yourself in the mirror with your hands on your hips and lean forwards and backwards and side to side

Figure 4.
Feel round each breast in a circular motion and then repeat with the other arm behind your head and check into the armpit (see fig 5)

Figure 5.

(for men only)

What should I be aware of?
- all men and boys should be 'testicle aware' - just as women are taught to be 'breast aware'
- testicular cancer is not a sexually transmitted infection
- it is seen mostly in young men
- the incidence of testicular cancer is on the increase
- cancer of the testicles has the highest treatment success rate of all cancers, so do not panic if you think there is a problem
- many other conditions, apart from cancer, cause swellings or lumps, so it is essential that you let a Doctor check you quickly - even if you may be embarrassed. This will ensure you get the correct diagnosis and treatment

What causes it?
the cause of testicular cancer is not proven but the main factors which may increase your risks are:
- your age - the highest risk group being 15 to 35 years olds
- if you had undescended testicles when you were born and needed an operation to bring one or both of them down into your scrotum
- trauma / accident / injury to the testicles

How often should I check?
- about once a month

How do I check them?
- it is a good idea to check your testicles, when the scrotum (skin sac) is relaxed
- in the bath or the shower is ideal
- as you check your testicles you will notice various lumps and bumps - consider these to be your guide and be on the 'look-out' for any change
- rest your testicles in the palm of your hand, to notice their weight and size
- you will probably notice that one testicle is larger than the other and may also hang lower than the other one - this is quite normal
- then gently roll each testicle, in turn, between your thumbs and fingers
- feel right round each one and up into the groin, behind them
- you will notice a 'spermatic cord' behind each testicle (a long, thin, round, semi-hard area, not a lump, as such)
- look at your testicles in the mirror and notice any visible changes

What else should I look for?
you may notice:
- a dull ache in the groin or abdomen
- heaviness in the scrotum
- occasionally there may be pain in the testicle itself

What if I notice something?
- first, check to see if it is on the other testicle, too
- if it is, it is extremely unlikely to be cancer, as it rarely develops on both sides at the same time

Now what do I do?

❖ make an appointment to see a Doctor

What if I've got cancer?

❖ this may sound drastic, but simple removal of the affected

I won't look 'normal' any more!

❖ the Doctors will probably discuss testicular implants with you, so you 'look' as you did before
❖ ask them for further information

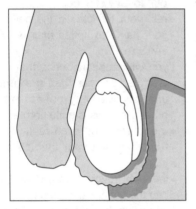

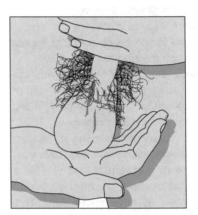

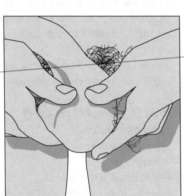

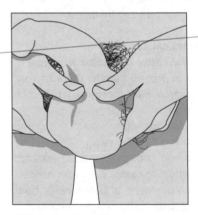

testicle when caught early, is usually all that is required
❖ the Doctors may decide to follow this up with special drug or x-ray treatment afterwards
❖ there is an *excellent* cure rate when the disease is caught and treated early

What about sex?

❖ you will be able to continue your sex life as before
❖ the other testicle will still be producing millions of sperm so your 'virility' and 'fertility' (ability to have sex and ability to be a father) should not be affected

* many people have infections without realising, **so this guide aims to protect you from all sexually transmitted infections - not just HIV**

FACT:

* in the tiny amount of blood involved in a 'needle stick injury' (syringe stab) the chance of getting HIV (if it is present) is 0.3%
* **BUT** the chance of getting hepatitis (if it is present) is 30% = 100 times more likely

Think about this!

* Doctors, Nurses, Surgeons and Dentists take 'universal precautions', (wear latex gloves) to protect themselves and treat all patients the same - i.e. as if there is a risk of infection
* is it not sensible to assume the same unknown risk when you have sex, and protect yourself - as they both involve contact with the blood or body fluids of another person?
* certain sexual activities take place without being spoken about openly, so this groups them at their most dangerous, for the risk of infection

* the **'safest sex'** is 'no sex' but that may be unrealistic!

'safer sex' *is the same for everyone - whether you are :* -

* **'straight'** - a man sexually attracted to women or a woman sexually attracted to men - heterosexual
* a **'gay man'** - a man sexually attracted to other men - homosexual
* **'lesbian'** - a woman who is sexually attracted to other women
* **'bisexual'** - someone who is sexually attracted to both men and women

'highest risk activities' include:-

* vaginal or anal sex without a condom, including 'coitus interuptus' (withdrawal)
* giving oral sex to a man (fellatio) if his ejaculate (also known as come / cum / semen / fluid / juice) enters your mouth
* giving oral sex to a woman (cunnilingus) during her 'period'
* unprotected 'rimming' (anilingus) - licking your partner's anus
* finger insertion if there are cuts, sores or menstruation
* SCAT - eating the human waste of another person
* drinking the urine of another person
* sharing sex toys
* unprotected group sex or group sex without a fresh condom for each 'partner change'

Sexplained © 1995 Helen Knox

'medium risk activities' include:-

❖ vaginal or anal sex with a condom

❖ giving oral sex to a man but not taking his ejaculate into your mouth

❖ oral sex with a man, but using a condom

❖ giving oral sex to a woman with her period, but using a barrier as protection between yourself and her body fluids (see 'oral sex & dental dams')

❖ giving oral sex to a woman - not during her period

❖ 'rimming' (licking your partner's anus) with the protection of a barrier (see 'oral sex and dental dams')

❖ **'wet' kissing** - (deep French kissing) depends upon the health of your and your partner's lips and mouth - i.e. bleeding gums (or newly brushed teeth when gums bleed), cut lips, 'cold sores' (herpes simplex), mouth ulcers etc. increase the risk, as hepatitis can easily pass this way and can be present in saliva. *You may prefer to suck a mint to freshen your breath, than brush your teeth before kissing another person*

❖ **foreplay and finger insertion** - if cuts, sores etc. are covered or if latex gloves are worn

Sex toys

❖ it is best to have your own personal sex toys (dildos/vibrators) but if you share them - the batteries should be removed and the 'toys' washed in hot soap and water then dried before use, and covered with a condom

❖ the condom should be changed for each person using the 'toy'

❖ the condom should also be changed if you go from anus to vagina with the 'toy' - otherwise there is a **high risk** of bowel germs entering the womb & tubes etc.

'low risk activities' (from the infection 'point of view') and <u>alternatives</u> to penetrative sex include:-

❖ masturbating your partner - but if any part of your hands enter their body it is sensible to make sure that **cuts, rashes or sores** are covered - either by a waterproof plaster or by latex gloves (condoms for hands!)

❖ masturbation - on your own

❖ the use of personal sex toys - but make sure they are washed in hot soapy water before and after use, each time

❖ kissing

❖ body kissing - of erogenous zones, such as ears, neck, breasts, abdomen, buttocks, toes etc.

❖ hugging

❖ sensual body massage

Note: if you use massage oils or body moisturising oils they **<u>must</u>** be fully washed off the penis with soap and water, before using a latex/rubber condom - or the rubber may rot and the condom will very likely break!

- body rubbing (frottage)
- corporal punishment - whipping and caning (with consent), as long as blood is not drawn (although, in law, this is assault)
- 'S&M' - sadomasochism - sexual excitement from inflicting or thinking of inflicting pain on another person, or getting sexual pleasure from experiencing pain or humiliation yourself (unless blood is drawn)
- general or erotic fantasy, using your own imagination or that of another in magazines, films, erotic and literature etc.
- dressing up - 'stockings & suspenders', 'uniforms' etc.
- stroking skin with different fabrics - silk, chiffon, leather and lace etc.
- love bites (as long as blood is not drawn)
- 'golden showers' / 'water sports' (urinating over your partner) as long as there are no open sores or cuts
- telling each other your erotic fantasies and 'role-playing' them together
- sexual arousal fully clothed - and remaining so!
- slow striptease to music with dim lighting etc.
- 'dirty' pillow talk to each other
- food! - licking your favourite food off your partner e.g. cream, champagne etc.
- anything else you can think of which doesn't involve the exchange of body fluids and gives **mutual** pleasure, by

consent/with permission

When should the male condom be used?

- there are approximately 300,000 sperm at the tip of an erect penis, which are enough to cause pregnancy and/or pass germs, in the right conditions, **without even penetrating (entering)** your partner
- therefore it is vital that the condom is used **_before_** there is **any genital contact** _whatsoever_ with your partner

How should the male condom be used?

both_ **men and women** should be competent in the skill of **'rolling on responsibility'**

- first, it is very important that if you have been using massage or other oily moisturisers on your penis, these must be washed off with soap and water before the condom is put on - otherwise there is a risk that the condom may rot/burst/split when it comes into contact with the oil (This is a common cause of condom failure)
- next follow these instructions carefully
- check the expiry date on the packet and that it conforms to recognised standards i.e. is the box marked with the British Standards 'kite mark', similar European ("CE") mark or international standard of the country you are in?
- check the wrapping has not been tampered with (damaged), before taking a condom from the packet

- gently tear the wrapping to expose the condom - **do not** use your teeth!
- look at it, or feel it, to check which way round it is going to unroll - the roll should be outwards
- check the 'teat' is easy to hold or if it does not have a 'teat', make your own, by squeezing the top one inch of the condom free of any air
- take the condom from its wrapping and ensure that you place the rolled up condom onto a fully erect penis
- **unroll** the condom downwards and over the penis for at least two inches **before** letting go of the 'teat'
- this ensures that no air slips back into the 'teat' (if it does, the condom may burst)
- continue unrolling the condom onto the penis until the whole of the penis is covered by it (right to the pubic hair line)

during sex

- it is sensible to check that the condom has not slipped slightly, as if it is coming off
- this is usually noticed by a slight change in sensation
- if it has, then just guide it back down the shaft of the penis and continue
- re-lubricate as necessary, or the condom may weaken if it gets too dry and the recipient will become sore from dry friction

after ejaculation

- ❖ ensure that the condom is held on the penis during withdrawal and that this happens before the penis starts to go 'soft'
- ❖ if not and you have 'gone soft', there is a greater chance that it may be gripped by your partner's muscles, slip off and spill inside them
- ❖ that would mean it was a waste of time and effort using the condom - risking pregnancy and/or infection!
- ❖ **use condoms once *only***

What if I make a mistake and put it on upside down?

- ❖ ***throw it away immediately***
- ❖ ***do not turn it over and try again***
  - because germs and sperm would be transferred *right inside your partner*, risking pregnancy and / or infection
- ❖ if that was your last condom - don't risk having unprotected sex and be more organised next time!

if anything does go wrong - remember that **'emergency contraception'** is available (see 'contraceptive tips')

'It bursts, it leaks, it doesn't feel the same' - why?

- ❖ if your partner is not sufficiently moist, the condom will 'dry out' making it sore to use and more likely to burst
- ❖ if you have oil on your penis, it can interact with rubber and the condom is likely to rot/

burst/split/break

What if I don't get all of the air out of the 'teat' when I put the condom on?

- ❖ it is said to be a contributing factor when condoms fail
- ❖ the pressure of ejaculation against the trapped air is thought to weaken the rubber and the condom may be more likely to 'burst/split' along the shaft of the penis - rendering its use ineffective

What if I have long nails / hang nails/ rough nails?

- ❖ these could easily puncture the rubber, so be very careful

'Condoms are too small for me, so I don't wear them'

- ❖ changing to a thinner condom in which the 'ring' is not as tight, should make the condom more comfortable to wear
- ❖ there is now a huge range of condoms to choose from - try various brands *until you find one to suit **you***
- ❖ *they come with short teats, long teats or no teats, straight sides, flared sides, baggy tips or tight fit, with or without spermicide, with or without lubricant, various colours and flavours, various thickness', - different lengths and* **'allergy condoms'** *- so try them all until you find what suits **you***
- ❖ with the introduction of the new European standard ('CE') condoms will be 10mm (1cm -

just under $^1/_2$") longer and range in width from 44mm - 56mm

'Condoms are too big for me, what should I do?'

❖ there are smaller and tighter condoms available now

❖ if you are young and they are too big for you, perhaps you should wait until you have fully grown before you have sex and you are physically mature

❖ there are condoms on the market to accommodate all sizes of mature penis

Some men suggest:

❖ try thicker condoms, if you feel that 'premature ejaculation' (coming too quickly) is a concern for you

❖ try tighter/smaller condoms if you notice a delay in ejaculation - they may help you 'come' (ejaculate) more easily

What if I feel I am allergic to condoms ?

❖ there are 'allergy' or 'hypo-allergenic' condoms available

❖ it may not be the condom, as such, but the lubricant on it

❖ try changing from condoms lubricated with spermicide (nonoxynol 9 or 11) to just lubricated condoms

❖ use a lot of extra 'water based lubricant' incase the 'allergy' is a friction based problem, from being too dry, which makes sex very uncomfortable

❖ try 'jel-charging' the condom, too

(see 'jel charging')

What is spermicide?

❖ it is a chemical to kill sperm

If I wear two condoms I'll be 'double safe', won't I?

❖ no, you won't

❖ they are more likely to fail/burst/split if used that way - instead, use the 'extra strong' varieties and a lot of water based lubricant.

❖ dispose of condoms after use by tying a knot at the open end and wrap it in a tissue, then throw in the bin

❖ do not try and flush used condoms in the loo - they tend to float!

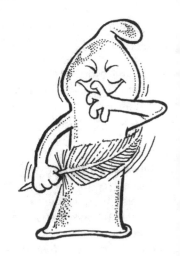

Which condom can I use for anal sex?

- ❖ no condoms are licenced for anal sex, as there are no 'anal sex' standards to which they can be tested
- ❖ but extra strong / ultra strong / 'industrial' varieties are slightly thicker and when used with a lot of water based lubricant, are best for this

As anal sex is the highest risk sex, how can I make it as safe as possible?

- ❖ this is still a taboo subject despite the fact that it is widely practiced, world-wide, by both men and women
- ❖ it became legal on April 9th 1995 in the UK, between concenting men and women over 18 years of age
- ❖ it was already legal between concenting men over 18 years of age
- ❖ some couples use it as a form of contraception
- ❖ some couples prefer to do it when the woman has her period
- ❖ it should NEVER be forced as this would be excruciatingly painful
- ❖ the anus is a very tight band of muscle which needs plenty of lubricant and arousal as it does not 'self-lubricate' or relax like the vagina to accommodate a finger, dildo or penis
- ❖ a finger, dildo or penis should never go from anus to vagina, as

the risk of bowel germs being passed to the vagina, womb, tubes etc. is very high this way

- ❖ always use a condom
- ❖ change condoms or wash thoroughly before vaginal sex

- ❖ the main forms of anal sex include - **anilingus or 'rimming'** (licking your partner's anus) - safest when using a dental dam - see 'oral sex and dental dams'
- ❖ **touching** or **'fingering'** - safest with a condom over the finger or wearing latex gloves, with water based lubricant
- ❖ **anal penetration -**
- by finger (see above)
- by sex toy - safest when washed first, then covered with a fresh condom each time and washed again after use
- by penis - a strong condom should always be used
- by fist - latex gloves and a lot of water based lubricant should always be used

Are there any effects from anal sex?

- ❖ in the 'short term' - the back passage may be torn, bleed slightly and cause constipation (from fear of the pain of opening the back passage after anal sex)
- ❖ if 'hepatitis A' is present, it can be passed by 'rimming'
- ❖ 'piles' may be more common
- ❖ 'fistulas and fissures' (tears and splits) to the anal area can occur

due to constipation, infection and/or because the area is repeatedly stretched

* if practiced 'long term', it can lead to damage of the tight band of muscle which keeps the back passage closed, the 'recipient' may become 'incontinent of faeces' and unable to control their 'flatulence/wind' (i.e. lose bowel control)

* with repeated stretching the anal sphincter can go into 'spasm' during anal sex and 'lock' the penetrative partner to the recipient

* as 'anal fisting' involves penetrating past the anal sphincter into the rectum/bowel (where there are fewer nerves to warn of pain) there can be more damage to (or tearing of) the bowel lining than might be realised (or felt) at the time, than if 'pain messages' could be relied upon to warn about 'internal damage'

for any type of anal sex:-

* never let anyone force you to have anal sex if you don't want to

* if you do indulge in anal sex make sure you do it as *safely* as possible

* **always** use condoms and a *lot* of water based lubricant to lubricate an otherwise dry area and prevent 'cross infection', friction sores and damage

* nails should always be kept short to avoid scratching the delicate tissue of the back passage

* if 'fingering or fisting', latex gloves should **always** be worn to prevent cross-infection, as the bowel has many germs within it

* be honest if you need medical care afterwards, for any reason

---

* **(beware** - 'poppers' act as a muscle relaxant, *but* affect the 'cardio-vascular' system, reduce blood pressure, induce headaches, shortness of breath, nausea, cold sweats, facial dermatitis and in excess, haemorrhage, collapse, coma and death!)

- in the context of a long term, loving, trusting, totally monogamous (one long-term partner) relationship, where each partner has been fully tested for any STD's before having sex together, oral sex is considered to be fairly safe
- the risks of germs passing, either way are, however, still there, although minor (e.g. NSU)
- oral sex in a casual or unfaithful relationship raises the risk considerably (oral gonorrhoea, herpes, syphilis, warts, etc.)
- hence the concept of 'dental dams'
- flavoured condoms are recommended for giving oral sex to a man
- Hepatitis 'B' and 'C' can be present in blood and body fluids and is 100 times easier to catch than HIV
- good personal hygiene is advisable before oral sex (e.g. washing the 'private areas')

Dental dams for oral sex! - what are 'dental dams'?

- originally they were sheets of 6 inch by 6 inch latex (rubber) used by Dentists, on patients mouths, but someone tried using them as barrier protection for oral sex
- they are placed over the whole 'private area' of a woman or the anal area of a man before they receive oral sex (anilingus)
- at present, they are expensive, should be used once only and do not have a 'use this way up' sign

on them - so you might like to mark it yourself
- otherwise, if it falls off and you replace it without checking, you could put it back the wrong way round - which defeats the object of using it in the first place!
- alternatively, make your own - by cutting a flavoured condom from base to tip and opening it up, to make a latex barrier (some people use 'cling film')
- using water based lubricant between a 'barrier' and the genitals increases sensation

Are there flavoured lubricants for oral sex?

- yes, there are
- they are available from specialist condom outlets
- your local Pharmacist may also be able to help you
- if you 'make your own' be careful not to use foodstuffs which have an oily base, as they will damage rubber/latex condoms

Where can I buy 'latex gloves' and / or 'dental dams?

- a Pharmacist can order them for you if they are not openly on display
- latex gloves are used for many other things, so you do not have to worry that the shop assistants will know why you want them

Sexplained © 1995 Helen Knox

- this is when a small amount of water based lubricant is put *inside* the tip of a condom before it is put on
- the air should still be expelled carefully from the top one inch as the condom is rolled over the penis
- massage the end of the condom so that the lubricant then covers the 'helmet' / 'knob' of the penis
- the extra moistness of 'jel charging' is said to greatly *increase sensation* - especially for **circumcised men**
- **uncircumcised men** should hold their foreskin right back before putting a condom on and may not require as much lubricant to enhance sensation
- some men state that 'jel charging' is *'wetter and better than sex without a condom'*
- your partner should also be regularly lubricated to avoid the condom 'drying out' and breaking when 'thrusting' for a long time
- **'jel charging'** may seem like a 'bit of a drag' but if it is built into foreplay can be an added enjoyment - especially if the sensation is improved by doing it!
- beware *in case* the condom slips more easily - due to the increased internal lubrication

What about 'Femidom®' the female condom?

- this is a fairly new contraceptive
- it looks as if it is a cross between a 'cap' and a loose condom
- as with the male condom - it is meant to be used once only
- it is made of 'polyeurethane' and is already lubricated
- it is inserted into the vagina, either by the woman or her partner
- part of it stays outside and covers the 'private area'
- it covers the clitoris - making oral sex safer
- an advantage of 'Femidom' is that **any** lubricant can be used with it - even 'oil based' ones, which damage rubber male condoms
- another advantage is that the man can keep his penis inside his partner after ejaculating - when his penis goes 'soft' (which he shouldn't do when using rubber male condoms)
- with the rubber/latex male condom he has to withdraw whilst still 'hard', holding the condom in place as he comes out - otherwise it may slip off, stay inside and spill - making it a waste of time and effort to have used it that time!
- a disadvantage is the price. They are more expensive than the male condom but FREE at some Family Planning Clinics

What if we always have 'safer sex' then don't want to bother, or want to have a baby?

- as you will want to know you are safe from getting any infections, the only sure way is for both of you to be fully tested at a GUM/STD Clinic before you have unprotected sex
- this still means you will have to trust that your partner is not having sex outside your relationship (even with a condom, as they can fail or come off, infections can be caught orally and anally too, putting you at risk when they have sex with you again)
- confidentiality is 100% at a GUM/STD Clinic and your GP is not informed unless you request this to happen

What about artificial insemination?

- sperm (and donors) at clinics specialising in this type of 'assisted fertility' is tested for HIV and the donor is re-tested 3 months after donating sperm - which is only used if the second test is also negative
- sperm donated by a male 'friend' for this purpose may put you 'at risk' unless the person has been fully tested and counselled about any legal implications of donating sperm
- 'one night stands' to become pregnant involve 'high risk sex' and are not advised at all

Are there any new male condoms?

- yes, plastic ones are available in the USA and planned for the UK soon
- they are more expensive than rubber latex condoms
- greater sensitivity is expected
- the main advantage of a plastic condom is that any lubricant can be used with it - oil based or water based
- with latex rubber condoms it is essential that only water based lubricants are used - or the rubber will rot in hardly any time - putting you 'at risk'!
- work is also under way on a 'super-latex'

Some general points to remember

- there is a risk of contracting infections with oral sex if it is 'unprotected', as germs do travel this way
- if you get a **sore throat after oral sex**, don't be shy to admit this to your Doctor, so they can treat you properly
- vaginal sex - after anal sex - is dangerous from the infection point of view, unless you use a condom and change it before entering the vagina
- vaginal sex BEFORE anal sex is safer if the condom cannot be changed

Sexplained © 1995 Helen Knox

Some people may 'find out' that their partner is bisexual (also has sex with their own sex) or that their partner is visiting 'sex workers'-

❖ these two situations have potentially serious health risks - both physically and emotionally

❖ people worried about this situation are advised to seek comprehensive medical 'check-ups' at a GUM/STD Clinic and may feel the need of support from their GP, Practice Nurse or Counsellor

❖ Family Planning Clinics have Nurses trained to support people through these situations

❖ GUM/STD Clinics also have counsellors and Health Advisors able to help

DO NOT USE with rubber male condoms or 'the cap' (diaphragm)

margarine
butter
low-fat spreads
ice cream
salad cream / mayonnaise
cooking oils
suntan oil
lipstick
body oil
cold cream
baby oil
cocoa butter
massage oil
Nivea
skin softener
hair conditioner
Vaseline
petroleum jelly
olive oil
engine oil!
hand cream
some soaps

❖plus *anything else which requires soap and water to wash it off your hands*

❖*where there is a risk of hepatitis* saliva *should* not *be used as a lubricant*

❖**remember - NEVER use Vaseline, petroleum jelly or oils with rubber condoms**

DO NOT USE these vaginal and rectal preparations with male rubber condoms and 'the cap' (diaphragm)

Arachis oil enemas
Baby oil
Cyclogest
Ecostatin
Fungilin
Gyno-daktarin
Gyno-pevaryl
Monistat
Nizoral
Nystan cream
Petroleum jelly
Nystavescent
Orthodienoestrol
Orthogynest
Pimafucin cream
Rendel pessaries
Sultrin
Vaseline
Witepsol based suppositories
Zinc and Castor oil

❖plus *anything else which requires soap and water to wash it off your hands*

❖**Women - please note!**
if you wear nail polish and you put a spermicidally lubricated condom (or with nonoxynol 9 or 11 written on the box) onto your partner or use spermicide with your 'cap' - your nail polish may soften

Sexplained © 1995 Helen Knox

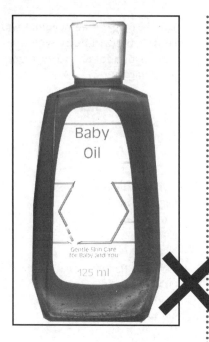

It is **OK to use the following vaginal and rectal preparations** with rubber condoms or 'the cap' (diaphragm)

aqueous enemas
Aci-jel
Boots lubricating jel
Betadine
Canesten
Clotrimazole
Comfort jel
Delfen foam
Delfen cream
Double-check
Durex Duragel
Durex Duracreme
Durex lubricating jel
Durex **Senselle**
Emko-foam
Glycerine
Gynol II
K-Y jelly
Liquid silk
Nyspes
Nystan pessaries (not cream)
Pearce jel
Sutherland Health jel
Replens
Staycept jelly
Staycept pessaries
Travogyn vaginal tablets
Travogyn cream
Two's Company
'Wetstuff'

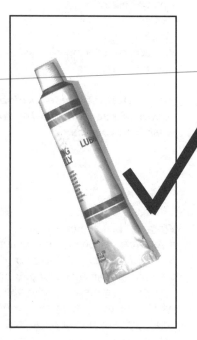

❖ **Many** other preparations are available from specialist condom outlets but - *always check before using any product*

- would your partner tell you if they had a 'one night stand', an affair, had sex with a 'sex worker', were raped, or had sex with anyone except yourself? - maybe - maybe not
- the honest answer is that you simply do not know, you can only hope they care enough about you and your health to tell you, before they have sex with you again and risk your life by their indiscretion
- many people in marriages, living together or simply 'going steady', be they straight, gay, lesbian or bisexual, know they are HIV positive, but are still prepared to put their partner 'at risk' and assume it is o.k. to have unprotected sex with them, because they are their 'regular' partner
- perhaps they are more scared of rejection than of protecting their partner - but how would they feel if they were the 'regular' partner?
- maybe they feel guilty and don't know how to tell their partner, but:
- a woman is many times more likely to catch HIV from a man than a man is from a woman
- most **men** get HIV from one night stands
- most **women** get HIV in *long term relationships!!!!*
- *you only ever really know your own sexual history*

- if you are a virgin and your partner is also a virgin you are just having sex with the germs of one person
- but, if you are a virgin and your first partner has had sex with 5 people - you are having sex with the germs of a minimum of **6** people (5 plus your partner)
- if you change partners (your 2nd partner) and use the same theory, you have sex with the germs of a minimum **30** people (their 5 partners and the 5 each of their partners have had)
- your 3rd partner = the germs of a minimum **155** people
- change again - your 4th partner = the germs of a minimum **780** people
- 5th partner change = **3,905**
- 6th partner change = **19,530**
- 7th partner change = **97,655**
- 8th partner change = **488,280**
- 9th change = **2,441,405**
- 10th change = **12,207,030**
- **plus all the people, all those other people, have had sex with too etc., etc.!!!!**

How do I negotiate having 'safer sex' when we haven't been using condoms and have been together a long time?

❖ some women are advised to change from other methods of contraception to condoms for medical reasons

❖ there are times when a woman taking the contraceptive pill needs to use extra protection (see 'tips' section)

❖ many simply want a rest from the responsibility of birth control and want to pass this to their partner

❖ one great advantage of condoms, is that the recipient (and the furniture, etc.) stays drier after sex, as the ejaculate is removed within the condom

❖ furthermore, it is now routine practice for Family Planning staff to recommend a 'double Dutch' approach - i.e. condoms plus another method of birth control

❖ **or** the use of condoms plus the routine use of extra spermicide

❖ this is a question you have to discuss together and examine your reasons for asking, very honestly

❖ you could just say that this is what you want to do, from now on, but how might your partner react?

❖ what might this question mean if they asked it of you?

❖ might it mean "I don't trust that you are faithful to me"

❖ **or** "I want to be unfaithful and use condoms with you, too, just incase I do catch anything and bring it back"

❖ **or** "it's a good idea, just in case either of us is unfaithful"

❖ **or** "I do trust you and hope you trust me, but if we use condoms routinely, you'll have more peace of mind and feel safer. I'd like us to use them, so I can relax and feel that you feel safer, with me"

❖ **or** do you make an absolute promise to each other, to remain faithful and be honest with each other, if either of you is unfaithful?

❖ **or** do you go together for a full STD check-up and realise the full implications of unfaithfulness, have an equal fear of the other's potential for being unfaithful and let that fear keep you faithful, because of how you would feel, if they were unfaithful to you and put your health at risk?

❖ how many people assume that it is alright to have 'unsafe sex' with their *regular partner* but have 'safer sex' with a *casual partner* - thinking this is all the precaution necessary to keep their 'secret' safe and undiscovered?

❖ **even the best of condoms can fail or be used incorrectly meaning that 'safer sex' was actually 'unsafe sex'!**

❖ not all sexually transmitted infections have instant signs or symptoms - but can 'ruin' the good thing you had, when your partner realises they have been cheated, deceived and their health put 'at risk'!

* the **only** *'safer sex'* is - *full* STD check-up before you have sex together then TOTAL FAITHFULNESS or NO SEX!
* unfaithfulness includes sex with male or female 'sex workers', 'bisexual' or casual 'gay' sex, having several 'regular' sexual partners, or indulging in 'group sex'

Some contraceptive tips for men and women

emergency contraception

* the new name for 'the morning after pill' is **'emergency contraception'/ 'emergency pills'**
* that is because the 'emergency pills' work, not just 'the morning after' but any time up to 72 hours (three days) after unprotected sex two special pills are taken by the woman, as soon as possible - followed by another two special pills, 12 hours later
* they are not, yet, given out in advance, but can be obtained from ALL Family Planning Clinics, most GP's, some hospital casualty departments and 'GUM/STD' clinics
* at the GP's you may have to tell the receptionist why you need an EMERGENCY appointment - otherwise they may say you cannot be seen until it is too late to prescribe the pills!
* some private clinics offer it too, but you have to pay a fee - look in the local phone book for information under 'Family Planning'
* if you are not suitable for, or unable to get, the 'emergency pill' within 72 hours, an **emergency IUD** or 'coil' can be inserted up to 5 days after unprotected sex
* most women would have had a period within three weeks from taking 'emergency pills' - if you have a lighter bleed than usual or

no bleed, see your Doctor to check and rule out an 'ectopic' (tubal) pregnancy

the combined pill (C.O.C.)

❖ if you are using the **combined oral contraceptive pill** (the pill) do you know when your protection is considerably reduced - perhaps lost?

❖ 'the pill' should be taken at the same time every day

❖ this ensures that a steady level of the hormones filters into the bloodstream, to keep the ovaries (where the eggs are made) asleep - thereby ensuring that you cannot get pregnant

❖ it is logical - no egg, no pregnancy

❖ **if, however, the pill is missed - but it is remembered within 12 hours from the time it should be taken, just take it as soon as you remember and you do not lose protection**

❖ **if you are over 12 hours from your usual pill taking time - your protection is lost**

❖ **in this case - do not stop the pills**

❖ **continue as usual, but use extra protection i.e. the condom, cap or no sex(!) for the next 7 days**

❖ **IF those 7 days go into what would have been your 7 day break between packets - do not take the break but start a new packet and take it to the end of the course (as usual)**

❖ then, at the end of that packet, have the break as usual

❖ taking two packets, 'back to back' will not harm you

❖ again, this explanation is logical - during the seven day break the ovaries start to 'wake up' and if they are not sent 'back to sleep' in time, there is the risk of an egg being released

❖ many people think that it takes several months to re-start releasing eggs after coming off 'the pill' - but this is *not* true

❖ if a woman has bad diarrhoea, vomiting, is taking **ANTIBIOTICS** or some other prescription medicines - it is wise to assume that protection has been lost

❖ **EXTRA PROTECTION (or no sex) is required for ALL the time of any illness or medication AND for 7 days after**

❖ **ALSO - if any of that time goes into what would have been the 7 day break between packets, she should continue straight into the next packet after completing the present packet - take all of those in turn - and then have the break (as above)**

❖ if in doubt about which medicines cause problems, check with the Doctor who prescribed them, ring any Family Planning Clinic, or ask a Pharmacist in a chemist shop

the P.O.P. / mini-pill

❖ if you are using the progestogen only pill (P.O.P. / mini pill) - are you positive which 'rules' apply to you?

❖ are you positive it is the 'mini pill' and not a ' low dose combined oral contraceptive pill'?

* the P.O.P. or 'mini-pill' as it is known in Family Planning - is the one containing just one hormone - progestogen
* it works by thickening the mucus at the neck of the womb, so that sperm cannot swim through to meet an egg
* it also has an effect on the lining of the womb, which helps to prevent pregnancy
* the pills must be taken at exactly the same time **EVERY DAY** of the year - with **NO** break
* the P.O.P. may cause irregular bleeding or stop the periods

If you forget a mini-pill (POP), what should you do?

* if you remember **within three hours** from the time you have set yourself to take it regularly - just take it and continue as normal
* **but,** **if you have forgotten for more than three hours - continue taking the pill as normal, when you remember, but you need to use EXTRA PROTECTION or have NO SEX for 7 days afterwards, to be safe**
* as with the 'combined pill' - if you have had bad diarrhoea or vomiting this will reduce your protection
* **EXTRA PROTECTION is required during the time of illness, with some medication AND to be safe, for 7 days after you are better**
* if in doubt, ask your Pharmacist

* (Note: this rule changed from 48 hours extra protection in July 1993)

EITHER PILL

* if in doubt, check with any Family Planning Clinic or your GP
* use extra protection unless you are **reliably** informed that it is not necessary
* always take the pill you are late with, even if this means taking two pills on one day
* **don't take any risks**

CITY AND ISLINGTON
SIXTH FORM COLLEGE
283 - 309 GOSWELL ROAD
LONDON

Sexplained © 1995 Helen Knox

Further Information

The numbers of these organisations are correct at the time of publication.

HIV/AIDS

National AIDS helpline - free calls

in English	0800 567 123
in Bengali, Gujerati, Hindi, Punjabi and Urdu	0800 371 134
in Cantonese (Tues 6-10 pm)	0800 282 446
In Arabic (Thurs 6-10 pm)	0800 282 447
for those 'hard of hearing' (10 am-10 pm daily)	0800 521 361

they also have an up to date list of numerous organisations, including:-
Scottish, Welsh, Northern Ireland and International AIDS helplines

BHAN (Black HIV/AIDS network)	0181 7492828
Bisexual helpline - London (Tues & Wed 7:30-9:30pm)	0181 569 7500
Edinburgh (Thurs 7:30-9:30 pm)	0131 557 3620

The Landmark - support for people with HIV/AIDS and their carers
0171 678 6686
Lesbian and Gay Switchboard - open 24 hours -   0171 837 7324
London Lighthouse - services for people with HIV/AIDS and their carers
0171 792 1200
Mainliners (HIV positive drug user support agency)   0171 678 6686
The Terrance Higgins Trust - advice, counselling and education about
HIV/AIDS 52-54 Gray's Inn Road, London WC1X 8JU   0171 242 1010

Family Planning

UK Family Planning Association, 27-35 Mortimer Street, London W1N 7RJ
provides national contraceptive helpline, Family Planning and GUM/STD
clinic advice locally, education and mail order bookshop
0171 636 7866
Family Planning Sales - mail order condoms, lubricants etc. 01865 749333
British Pregnancy Advisory Service - BPAS - privately run charity offering
Family Planning, Well Woman, assisted fertility, abortion advice and
help   0171 222 0985
Pregnancy Advisory Service - PAS - similar to above   0171 637 8962
Brook Advisory Centres - contraception and advice centres for young men and
women under 25 years of age. Centre locations throughout the UK
0171 713 9000
Marie Stopes International - similar to BPAS and PAS   0171 388 4843

General information

Acceptance - advice and counselling for parents of lesbian and gay men
01795 661 463

Alone in London - information for people under 21, single and homeless
0171 278 4224

Beaumont Society - offers support for transvestities and transexuals
0181 756 1782

British Liver Trust - support and advice for people concerned about hepatitis
and other liver conditions   01473 276 362

Childline - advice and support for children   0800 11 11

Childline for children in care - lines open from 5-10 pm   0800 88 44 44

Consent - helps male survivors of sexual abuse and rape -
their families & friends   0171 613 5486

Herpes Association - supports people with or worried about herpes
0171 609 9061

Incest Crisis Line - offers support for people abused by ralatives
0181 890 4732

National Drugs Helpline - answers questions about drugs and
can refer you to local services   0800 77 66 00

Rape Crisis - offers support for victims of rape - 24 hours a day
0171 837 100

Sexwise - young people's helpline - open 7am to midnight 7 days a week
0800 282 930

S.P.O.D. - information / advice abour sexual problems of the disabled
0171 607 8851

T.I.N. - teenage information network - provides advice on sex, drugs, HIV,
STD's,contraception and testing for young people   0171 403 2444

Women's Reproductive Rights Information Centre   0171 251 6580

Knox Publishing
PO Box 6969
Chiswick
London W4 3WX

Mail order form for more copies of this book :
'Sexplained .... the uncensored guide to sexual health'
by Helen Knox

price £9:99 each
plus £1:50 post and packing in the UK
total UK mail order **price £11:49 each**
for orders abroad, please add £2:50 for post and packing
total overseas mail order **price £12:49 sterling, each**
(please allow 28 days for delivery)

Order Form

- cut here -

Customer details

Date:............................
Name:(in capital letters) ....

Address:(in capital letters)...

....

....

Post code: .... **Full contact telephone number**..

Please send me ....(number of copies) of your book **'Sexplained .... the uncensored guide to sexual health'** at the price of £9:99 plus post and packing, as above.

Number of copies	at £9:99 each	£.................
plus UK post and packing	at £1:50 per copy	£.................
or plus overseas post and packing	at £2:50 per copy	£.................

TOTAL price enclosed   **£**_____

Please
1.   make cheques payable to 'Knox Publishing'
2.   write your cheque card number on the back of the cheque
3.   write your address on the back of the cheque
4.   tick here if you do **not** want information about further publications sent to you ....
5.   print here if you would like the book dedicated to someone and what you would like quoted:

....
....
....

In addition, please state where you obtained this copy of
'Sexplained .... the uncensored guide to sexual health'

I obtained this copy from (name and address of person or shop)...
....
....

Thank you for your order and your help
Knox Publishing, PO Box 6969, Chiswick, London W4 3WX, UK